Ace the CCRN®!

You can do it!

Study Guide

Nicole Kupchik

MN, RN, CCNS, CCRN, PCCN, CMC

Nicole Kupchik Consulting, Inc.

Seattle, WA

Nicole Kupchik Consulting and Education

ISBN-10: 0-9978349-2-7

ISBN-13: 978-0-9978349-2-5

Cover design by O'Daniel Designs

Printed in the United States of America

Seattle, WA

www.nicolekupchikconsulting.com

Special thanks...

To my husband, Carl

My mom, Carol

My many awesome friends
(you all know who you are...)

Kristin Nathan

Kyla Woodward

Dr. Elizabeth Bridges, for your years of mentoring

Marilyn Richards

Karen Lynn Maher

Gina O'Daniel

My colleagues at Harborview & Swedish who
have always encouraged me over the years!

And the THOUSANDS of nurses who attended
my classes, gave constructive feedback and took
the exams! You are all an inspiration to me!

The encouragement you all have given me is
immeasurable and completely appreciated!

Foreword

The Institute of Medicine's landmark report the *Future of Nursing* issued a call for nurses to lead, including nursing leadership at the point of care.[1] While we often think about leadership as a position, it has another definition. **A leader is "an expert clinician, involved in providing direct clinical care, who influences others to continuously improve the care they provide."** [2]

One key aspect to providing this leadership is clinical expertise and the ability to use evidence to inform practice. Preparation for certification is more than the rote memorization of facts. It is about teasing out complex situations and identifying critical information to guide your practice. The process of preparing for certification will advance your knowledge, competence and understanding the complexities of critical care nursing. [3]

But equally important to the increase in overt knowledge, this process will have less obvious or conceptual effects, such as an increased awareness of the evidence that support your practice, an increased confidence in your ability and passion to use evidence culminating

---

[1] Institute of Medicine Committee on the Robert Wood Johnson Foundation Initiative on the Future of Nursing at IoM. The Future of Nursing: Leading Change, Advancing Health. Washington (DC): *National Academies Press* (US); 2011.

[2] Cook MJ. Improving care requires leadership in nursing. *Nurse Educ Today*. 1999;19(4):306-12.

[3] Sayre C, Wyant S, Karvonen C. Effect of a medical-surgical practice and certification review course on clinical nursing practice. *J Nurs Staff Dev*. 2010;26(1):11-6.

in the "aha" moments when concepts come to life. Ultimately this subtle and empowering use of evidence supports its more overt or instrumental use, to persuade others and to advocate for practice and policy change. [4][5]

How do these concepts apply to this book? *ACE the CCRN* is a book designed to help you gain knowledge and enhance your ability to interpret and respond to complex clinical situations. But this book is not just a resource to aid you in preparing for a certification examination. Rather it reflects the author's passion to support your development as an expert critical care nurse. Along the way, the process towards certification may enhance both your conceptual and instrumental use of evidence. Think back to the definition of leadership, this journey to certification is really a journey to leadership and the advancement of our profession, and that is exactly what Nicole Kupchik is committed to.

—Elizabeth Bridges
PhD, RN, CCNS, FCCM, FAAN

---

4   Nutley S, Walter I, Davies H. How research can inform public services. Bristol, UK: *The Policy Press*, 2007.

5   Wilkinson JE. *Impacts of evidence use-hard hitting or subtle change? Worldviews on Evidence-Based Nursing.* 2010;7(1):1-3.

Unless we are making
progress in our nursing
every year, every month, every week,
take my word for it,
we are going back.

—Florence Nightingale (May 1872)

Contents

A note of encouragement from Nicole...

Congratulations on taking steps to becoming certified and obtaining the CCRN®!

In 2002, I passed the CCRN® for the first time. I am going to let you in on a little secret. I was eligible to sit the exam in 1994. I attended three certification review courses before taking the exam. Why? I lacked confidence and was so afraid of failing. I finally got up the courage in 2002 and aced it!

I can distinctly remember walking out of the testing site questioning myself, wondering why I waited so long to take it. I had so much self-doubt. It was a little crazy, because clinically, I knew my stuff. A couple years later, I started teaching sections of the exam at Harborview Medical Center and in 2006 started co-teaching prep courses nationally.

Who would think someone could go from having a complete lack of confidence to teaching the courses a few years later?! Mental mindset is everything. I want you to tell yourself every day that you can do this!!!

I often hear nurses say "becoming certified doesn't make you a better nurse". I completely disagree with statements like that. The journey you will take in preparing to become certified increases your knowledge to better care for your patients. I truly believe every nurse should be certified in their specialty.

I was inspired to publish this book by nurses who have attended my review courses. Many of the study books available are overwhelming & contain too much information. My goal is always to break down disease states into digestible pieces so you learn! The book is written with the purpose of being succinct & easy to read with bullet point formatting.

My biggest piece of advice to you in studying is, of course to understand different conditions, but do as many practice test questions as possible. Read rationales for questions you get right & those you miss. Consider using Ace the CCRN®: You can do it! Practice Question Review book to assist. The book contains 3 full practice tests and all answers have rationales. I believe practicing test questions is the key to success!

You can do it!

Thank you to the following reviewers:

Kristin Nathan BSN, RN, CCRN

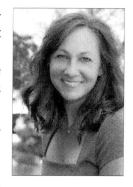

Kristin Nathan works as the clinical nurse educator in the Cardiovascular Intensive Care Unit at Legacy Emanuel Medical Center in Portland, Oregon. She earned her BSN from the Ohio State University and is currently pursuing her Masters in Nursing Education.

She has spent the past 18 years practicing as a critical care nurse and educator in Cardiovascular Medicine. She has held a position as a clinical adjunct faculty at Linfield Good Samaritan School of Nursing. She has spoken nationally promoting CCRN certification and has collaborated with the Greater Portland Chapter of AACN speaking for their statewide critical care nursing consortium.

Kyla F Woodward MN, RN, Alumnus CCRN, Alumnus PCCN

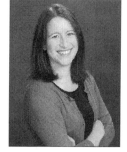

Kyla has 16 years of experience in nursing, with a clinical background in trauma and surgical critical care, progressive care, and stroke. After finishing her Master's, Kyla worked as a critical and progressive care educator in the hospital setting. She has taught a variety of clinical and classroom courses at Seattle hospitals and held a faculty role at the UCSF School of Nursing.

Kyla is passionate about nursing certification and has contributed to several certification review books and courses. She plans on returning to graduate school in the next few years to pursue a doctorate in nursing with a focus on education.

About the CCRN® Exam

The CCRN® is administered by the American Association of Critical Care Nurses (AACN). Website: www.aacn.org

Qualifications to sit the exam:

- Hold a current unencumbered nursing license

- Practice 1,750 hours in the previous 2 years

- 875 hours in the most recent year preceding application

- RNs or APRNs practicing for > 5 years with at least 2,000 practice hours, only need to work 144 hours in the most recent year

- If you have any questions about eligibility, please contact AACN—they are super helpful!

The application consists of 3 pages total. Two pages ask about demographic data, one page is an honor statement. You will need to provide the name & contact information of a colleague or manager who can verify your eligibility.

Once AACN receives your application, they usually take about 2 - 4 weeks to process everything. Once it has been processed & you are deemed eligible, you will receive an email and postcard from a company called AMP. They will give you directions to schedule your exam. You have 90 days to schedule. Easy peasy!

The CCRN® exam consists of 150 questions. Twenty five questions will not count toward your final score. They are used for statistical data for future exams. It's kind of a bummer that you don't know which ones don't count. The advice I ALWAYS give nurses—if you come across a question that you have NO idea the answer, tell yourself it's a question that doesn't count! Don't psych yourself out if you don't know the answer. There will be some questions that you just don't know.

Exam questions are written at the application & analysis levels based on Synergy model of care; meaning they aren't basic questions. They want to know you know how to take care of patients and what to anticipate in treatment. On that same thought, they also aren't trying to trick you. Each question will have 4 answer choices and only one is the correct answer.

You will have 3 hours to complete the exam. The passing "cut score" is 89. You have to get 89 correct out of 125. Translated—you have to score about 71% correct to pass. That's it!!! You can do this!!!! BUT, you have to go in prepared. In general, the reported pass rate for the CCRN® exam is about 74%. The way they score is a little more complicated than a straight 71%, but I'm not completely sure exactly how that's done.

THE CCRN® BLUEPRINT
NEW PLAN AS OF OCTOBER 15, 2015

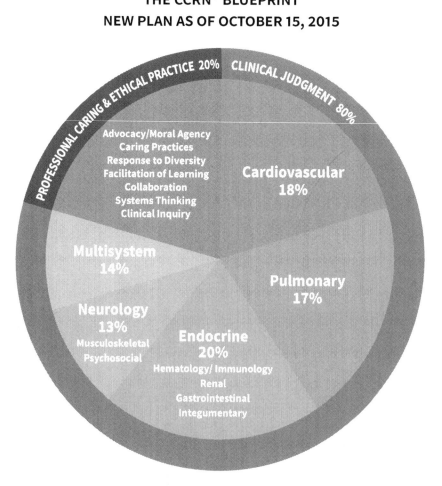

There is a newer exam called the CCRN®–K! ("K" stands for knowledge). It was initially offered September 2014. The exam is intended for nurses who have the critical care knowledge, but maybe don't work at the bedside as much. Eligible positions include clinical or patient educators, managers, administrators, academic faculty, etc.

Requirements for the CCRN®-K include:

* Current unencumbered licensure as an RN or APRN in the U.S.

* Practice as an RN or APRN for 1,040 hours within the previous two (2) years

* 260 of those hours accrued in the most recent year

GENERAL TEST TIPS:

✓ Go in with attitude! Confident attitude! You can do this!

✓ Get to the testing site on time

✓ Answer every question

✓ You can change answers, but...DON'T!!

✓ You'll have a clock in the lower right hand corner of your computer screen

✓ Pace yourself

✓ You will find out right away if you passed!

Positive Mental Attitude

Cardiovascular Review

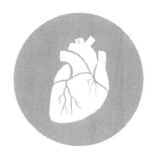

AACN Blueprint for the Cardiovascular portion of the CCRN© Exam

- Acute coronary syndromes/unstable angina
- Acute myocardial infarction & ischemia/papillary muscle rupture
- Acute peripheral vascular insufficiency (e.g., carotid artery stenosis, endarterectomy, fem-pop bypass, peripheral stents)
- Acute pulmonary edema
- Arterial-venous occlusion
- Cardiac catheterization (diagnostic & interventional)
- Cardiogenic shock
- Cardiomyopathies (e.g., dilated, hypertrophic, idiopathic, restrictive)
- Dysrhythmias
- Heart failure
- Hypertensive crisis
- Myocardial conduction system defects
- Structural heart defects (acquired & congenital, including valvular disease)
- Ruptured or dissecting aneurysm (e.g., thoracic, abdominal, thoraco-abdominal)

Coronary Artery Perfusion

» Both the right & left **coronary arteries** arise at the base of the aorta (Sinus of Valsalva); immediately above the aortic valve

» Coronary arteries are perfused during diastole

Heart Sounds

Valvular auscultation points:

» Aortic valve: Right sternal border, 2nd ICS

» Pulmonic valve: Left sternal border, 2nd ICS

» Tricuspid valve: Left sternal border, 4 - 5th ICS

» Mitral valve: Left mid-clavicular line, 5th ICS

Normal Heart Sounds

» S_1: closure of the mitral & tricuspid valves

* Loudest over mitral area, 5th ICS

* Systole

* 1/3 of the cardiac cycle

» S_2: closure of pulmonic & aortic valve

* Loudest over aortic area, 2nd ICS

* Diastole

* 2/3 of the cardiac cycle

Extra Heart Sounds

» S_3 : Ventricular gallop

* Auscultated in fluid overload; when preload is elevated

* Normal in kids, high cardiac output, 3rd trimester of pregnancy

* Listen over apex area

* Sound is caused by a rapid rush of blood into a dilated, overfilled ventricle

* Other causes: Cardiomyopathy, ventricular septal defect (VSD), mitral or tricuspid regurgitation

» S$_4$: Atrial gallop (pre-systolic)

- Sound caused by vibration of atria ejecting into non-compliant ventricles

- Auscultated during ischemia (increased resistance to ventricular filling)

- Other causes: Ischemia, HTN, pulmonary stenosis, CAD, aortic stenosis, left ventricular hypertrophy

- Listen over tricuspid or mitral area

» Split Heart Sounds

- When one valve closes later than the other

  ▷ **best heard during *inspiration*

- Split S$_1$—Mitral closes before tricuspid valve

  ▷ RBBB or PVC

- Split S$_2$—Aortic closes before pulmonic valve

  ▷ Overfilled right ventricle

  ▷ Atrial septal defect (ASD)

Acute Coronary Syndrome

Pathophysiology: Progressive atherosclerosis with plaque rupture causing blood clot formation leading to an imbalance of O$_2$ supply & demand

In ACS, there is an imbalance of oxygen supply & demand

O$_2$ Supply:

» Coronary arteries

» Diastolic filling time

» Cardiac output

» Hemoglobin

» SaO$_2$

O$_2$ Demand:

» Heart rate

» Contractility

» Preload

» Afterload

Cardiac Risk Factors

Non-modifiable:

- » Age
- » Gender
- » Family history
- » Race

Modifiable:

- » Smoking
- » Hyperlipidemia
- » Obesity
- » Diabetes mellitus
- » Diet
- » Physical inactivity
- » Hypertension

Cardiac Biomarkers:

- » Troponin I most sensitive & specific
- » Elevates in 3 - 6 hours
- » Peaks in 14 - 20 hours
- » Returns to normal in 1 - 2 weeks
- » Most labs > 0.4 mcg/L is considered elevated
- » CPK, CK-MB & myoglobin may also be elevated (no longer recommended to routinely check)

Unstable Angina & Non-ST Elevation MI (NSTE-ACS)

Chest pain assessment—ask these questions:

- » **O**nset?
- » **L**ocation?
- » **D**uration?
- » **C**haracteristics?
- » **A**ssociated s/s?
- » **R**elieving factors?
- » **T**reatment?

Angina

» Stable

* Exertional;
  pain goes
  away when
  exertion stops

» Unstable (UA)

* Increasing
  frequency,
  time,
  duration

* 10 - 20%
  have a MI

» Variant (Prinzmetal's)

* Sudden pain caused from
  coronary vasospasm

* Occurs at rest or when sleeping

* Get 12 lead ECG with
  & without pain!

* Will see ECG changes with
  pain and symptoms

* Treat with nitroglycerin
  (NTG), calcium channel
  blockers to relieve spasm

NSTE-ACS (NSTEMI)

» Partial occlusion of
coronary artery

» Pain/symptoms may occur
at rest & last > 20 min

» Hallmark sign—pain with ↑
frequency, heaviness or pressure

» 12 lead ECG: ST depression or
T wave inversion (ischemia)

» 8 or more leads with ST
depression/T wave inversion & ST
elevation in AVR, high suspicion
for proximal LAD occlusion

» Cardiac biomarkers elevated

» Treatment: PCI; early
PCI if high risk

ST Elevation MI (STEMI)

» Complete occlusion of
a coronary artery

» Emergency!

» 12 lead ECG: ST elevation
(infarction)

» Hallmark signs—Chest
pain or pressure > 20
min, SOB, diaphoresis

» Cause: Plaque rupture leading
to blood clot formation

* Platelets aggregate to
  the atherosclerotic site/
  plaque rupture

- Occlusive thrombus formation

» + Cardiac biomarkers

» Treatment: Immediate reperfusion

- Cath lab for PCI (preferred) or
- If Cath lab is not readily available—fibrinolytics, then Cath lab as soon as possible

ST depression = ischemia

ST elevation = injury

» ≥ 1 mm in limb leads (I, II, III, aVF, aVL) or ≥ 2 mm in precordial leads (V_1–V_6) and/or

» New left BBB precordial leads

» In 2 or more contiguous leads (leads that look at the same wall of the heart)

Timing of ECG Changes in STEMI:

» **Immediate:** ST ↑ in leads over the area of infarction

» **Within a few hours:** Large upright T waves

» **Several hours:** After revascularization, ST normalizes, T waves invert

» **Several hours–days:** Q waves may develop, reduced R waves, low voltage R wave (sometimes for life)

Emergent STEMI Treatment:

Aspirin

» 81 mg – 325 mg PO load

» Inhibits cyclooxygenase-1 within platelets → prevents formation of thromboxane A_2

» Disables platelet aggregation

» Monitor for intolerance

» Used indefinitely post MI

» Maintenance dose for life at least 81 mg daily

» Onset of action 1 – 7.5 min

Nitroglycerin

» 0.4 mg SL every 5 minutes x 3

» Sublingual, spray or
intravenous (Tridil)

» May use IV if continued
chest discomfort

» Potent vasodilator

» Monitor for hypotension,
headache

» Reduces preload &
ventricular wall tension

» Decreases myocardial
O_2 consumption

» Avoid if suspected right
ventricular infarction   Nitro

Supplemental O_2 only if sats < 94%

» Hyperoxemia perpetuates
oxidative injury after MI

» Can worsen and increase
infarct size with hyperoxemia

» Not needed for patients
without evidence of respiratory
distress (AHA guideline)

Morphine

» Small incremental doses
IV Q 5 - 15 min if chest pain
is unrelieved by NTG

» Use as adjunct therapy to NTG

» Potent analgesic & anxiolytic

» Causes venodilation &
reduces preload

» Decreases workload of heart

» Use cautiously in UA & NSTEMI!!

   • Increased mortality in a
   large patient registry

» Avoid if suspected right
ventricular infarction   Morphine

Post PCI therapy, consider:

» Access site management

- Radial artery access site is becoming more popular; fewer complications

- Femoral—monitor for bleeding, hematoma, retroperitoneal bleeding

» Retroperitoneal bleeding— will see "soft" BP that is fluid responsive

- Late sign is flank ecchymosis (Grey-Turner's sign)

- Assess coags

- Control bleeding

» Monitor renal function closely (secondary to dye load)

Post-PCI medication management:

Dual Anti-Platelet Therapy for at least 1 year post PCI

» **Aspirin** (indefinitely) **plus**

» **Thienopyridines** (P_2Y_{12} Inhibitors)—**with drug eluting or bare metal stents:**

- Clopidogrel (Plavix) 300 - 600 mg load; continue 75 mg daily for 12 months **or**

- Prasugrel (Effient) 60 mg load; continue 10 mg for 12 months **or**

- Brillinta (Ticagreolor) 180 mg load; 90 mg BID for 12 months

On a case by case basis, the cardiology provider may prescribe:

» Unfractionated Heparin (UFH) **or**

» Bivalirudin (Angiomax)—used during PCI; finish in Cath lab

» GP IIb/IIIa Inhibitors (at time of PCI)

- Abciximab (Reopro)

- Eptifibatide (Integrilin)

- Tirofiban (Aggrastat)

  ▷ Monitor platelet count

Beta Blockers: "-olols"

» Start within 24° if hemodynamically stable

» Hold if hypotension or signs of hypoperfusion/shock

» Metoprolol (Lopressor, Toprol XL) & carvedilol mostly used

» Blocks catecholamine & sympathetic nervous system

» Decreases HR & contractility

» Decreases myocardial O_2 consumption

» Long term, decreases morbidity & mortality

» Continued indefinitely

Statins (HMG CoA Reductase Inhibitors)

» ↓ cholesterol levels by interfering with body's ability to produce cholesterol

» ↓ inflammatory response that theoretically may be responsible for atherosclerotic process

» Statins recommended for all Post MI patients with:

- LDL cholesterol > 100
- atorvastatin (Lipitor), rosuvastatin (Crestor), lovastatin (Mevacor), simvastatin (Zocor)
- Monitor for myopathies & myositis

ACE Inhibitors ("prils") or Angiotensin Receptor Blockers ("sartans")

» EF < 40%, new heart failure

» Decrease intra-cardiac pressures

» Prevent cardiac remodeling

Common ACE Inhibitors:

» Ramipril (Altace), lisinopril (Zestril, Prinivil), enalapril (Vasotec), captopril (Capoten)

» Monitor for cough, angioedema, ↑ potassium, ↑ BUN & creatinine

Common ARBs:

» Valsartan (Diovan),
  losartan (Cozaar)

If cardiac catheterization/PCI is not available within 90 – 120 min, fibrinolytics may be considered.

Fibrinolytic Therapy

» Tenecteplase (TNKase) -
  fast rapid IV bolus or

» Activase (rtPA)

• Bolus followed by infusion

• Will still need to go to the
  Cath lab once bleeding
  risk is diminished

Indications:

» Pain < 6 hours

» ST elevation > 1 mm in 2 or
  more contiguous leads

Contraindications to fibrinolytics: (higher bleeding risk)

Absolute:

» Active bleeding

» Intracranial hemorrhage

» Known cerebral vascular lesion

» Ischemic stroke in last 6
  mos. (except acute CVA)

» Malignant intracranial neoplasm

» Suspected aortic dissection

» Closed head or facial
  trauma within 3 mos.

» A-V malformation

Relative:

» Chronic, severe, poorly tolerated HTN

» SBP > 180 mm Hg or DBP > 110 mm Hg (lower BP prior to administration)

» Ischemic CVA > 3 mos.

» Dementia

» Traumatic or prolonged CPR

» Major surgery (< 3 weeks)

» Internal bleeding (within 2 - 4 weeks)

» Pregnancy

» Active peptic ulcer disease

» Current use of anticoagulants

Nursing Considerations post fibrinolytic administration:

» Frequent neurological assessment (d/t bleeding risk)

» Avoid punctures

» Monitor urine output & BUN/creatinine

» Avoid invasive devices

» Avoid compressive devices

Discharge: Education, education, education!

» Medication adherence

» Minimize ETOH

» Smoking cessation

» Exercise

» Lose weight (if applicable)

» Heart healthy diet

» Lower cholesterol & lipids

» Stress reduction

Acute Coronary Syndrome & 12 Lead ECG

ECG: What do the waves represent?

» P wave: Atrial depolarization

» PR interval: AV conduction time (0.12 – 0.20)

» QRS: Ventricular depolarization (0.06 – 0.10)

» T wave: Ventricular repolarization

» QT Interval (0.36 – 0.44)

Q-waves—Considered pathologic if:

» Width > 30 ms (0.04)

» Depth ≥ 25% of the height of the R wave

» If present in contiguous leads, indicative of myocardial necrosis

12 Lead ECG Summary

Location	Change in lead:	Reciprocal changes in lead: (ST Depression)	Artery affected:	Notes:
Inferior	II, III, aVF	I, aVL	RCA in 65% L circumflex	Right sided ECG assesses V_2R - V_4R
Septal	V_1 - V_4	II, III, aVF	LAD	
Anterior	V_2 - V_4	II, III, aVF	LAD/L main	
Lateral	I, aVL, V_5 - V_6		L circumflex, LAD	
Posterior	Posterior leads V_{7-9}	V_{1-2}	L circumflex, RCA	Tall upright R wave
Right ventricle	V_2R - V_4R		Proximal RCA	

Types of Myocardial Infarctions

Inferior wall MI

» Occlusion of the right coronary artery (RCA)

» Elevation in leads II, III & aVF

• Reciprocal changes in Leads I & aVL

• Will see changes better in lead III vs. lead II

Symptoms:

» Bradycardia

» High grade AV heart blocks— may need temporary pacer

» First degree AV Block

» Second degree Type I (Wenckebach)

» Hypotension

» N/V

» Diaphoresis

» Monitor for signs of right ventricular infarction

Right Ventricular Infarction

» Associated with proximal RCA occlusion & inferior wall MI

» If right ventricular infarction is suspected, get a right sided ECG

• Move precordial leads to right side of chest

• If infarction, will see ST elevation in $V_2R - V_4R$

Symptoms:

» Tachycardia

» Hypotension

» + JVD (with clear lungs)

» ECHO—the RV is often stunned with poor wall motion; blood backs up on the right side

» Poor forward flow to the left side of the heart

Treatment:

» **IV fluids (maximize preload!)

» Use small boluses, titrate to effect

» + Inotrope (increase contractility) i.e. Dobutamine

Avoid medications that lower preload:

» Nitrates, morphine, beta blockers, diuretics

» RV is often stunned and becomes preload dependent

Anterior/Septal Wall MI

» Changes noted in V_1 - V_4

» Reciprocal changes in II, III, aVF

» Loss of R wave progression in the precordial leads (V_1 – V_6)

» Left anterior descending/ left main occlusion

Symptoms:

» Left ventricular failure (S_3 heart sound)

» Shock

» Heart block (2nd degree Type 2, 3rd degree)

» Bundle branch block

» If new loud murmur, suspect ventricular septal rupture or papillary muscle rupture

   • get an echocardiogram

Conduction defects with anterior wall MI:

» Second degree type II AV block

   • Block occurs below the AV node

   • Can progress to complete heart block (CHB)

   • Constant PR interval, QRS blocked

   • If 2:1 block, can be difficult to diagnose

   • Prepare to emergently pace!

» Complete heart block
(Third degree AV block)

- No atrial impulses pass
through the AV node

- Ventricles generate
their own rhythm

- Ventricular rate is often
slow—20s to 40s

- Prepare to emergently pace!

Lateral wall MI:

» Changes in V_5, V_6, I, aVL

» Occlusion of the left circumflex

» Can be associated with other MI
locations (inferior, anterior)

Posterior Wall MI:

» Reciprocal changes in V_1 - V_2

» Tall, broad R wave (> 0.04)
in V_1 - V_2 & ST depression
(reciprocal change)

» Consider a posterior ECG

- ST elevation in posterior
leads V_7 - V_9

- Leads follow path around
the chest wall

» Associated with inferior
or lateral wall MI

» Occlusion of RCA or
left circumflex

Complications of Acute Myocardial Infarction

Pericarditis

» Inflammation of the
pericardial sac

» Acute or chronic

» Chest pain—sharp,
stabbing, or dull & achy

» Pain improved when sitting
up, leaning forward

» Left sided radiation

» Pain worse with cough,
positional changes & inspiration

» Pericardial friction rub

Treatment:

» NSAIDS—high dose Ibuprofen

» Antibiotic if bacterial, antifungal if fungus

Papillary Muscle Rupture

» Clinical signs: associated w/ anterior wall MI:

* Hemodynamic instability

* New LOUD systolic murmur

* Acute MITRAL REGURG!!!

* Diagnosed by ECHO

* Large "v" waves in PAOP waveform

Treatment:

» Hemodynamic support

» Emergent surgical repair/ valve replacement

Ventricular Septal Rupture

» Associated with septal wall MI

» Oxygen rich blood shunts to the right side of the heart from the left

* "Left to right shunting"

» At risk: anterior/septal wall MIs

Symptoms:

» Acute SOB

» S_3 heart sound

» Crackles

» Holosystolic murmur

PA catheter insertion:

» Falsely elevated C.O. on PA Cath because C.O. is derived from the right ventricle (left to right shunting)

* Increased SvO_2 due to left to right shunting

* Large "v" waves in CVP waveform

Cardiogenic Shock

Clinical signs:

» S_3, +JVD, pulmonary edema

» Tachycardia

» Dysrhythmias

» Signs of decreased perfusion

» Decreased UOP (oliguria < 0.5 ml/kg/hr)

Hemodynamics:

» Hypotension (MAP < 65)

» CI < 2 L/min/m²

» SVR > 2000 dynes/sec/cm⁻⁵

» Elevated RAP/CVP

» ↑PAOP; > 18 mm Hg

» Decreased SvO_2 (< 65%)

Other diagnostics:

» ABG—Mixed respiratory & metabolic acidosis; hypoxemia
  * Lactic acidosis

» Chest x-ray: pulmonary congestion and edema

» Echo: decreased wall motion, reduced ejection fraction

» Supportive treatment:
  * Vasopressors to support blood pressure
  * + Inotrope (i.e. Dobutamine) to improve contractility
  * Loop diuretics (as perfusion allows, decrease preload)
  * Afterload reduction / venous vasodilators (i.e. NTG)
  * Mechanical support (i.e. IABP, Impella)

Pulmonary Edema

» Fluid in the alveolus

» Impaired gas exchange, hypercapnia

» Hypoxemia

» Treatment: loop diuretics

Pharmacologic Action and Target of Vasopressors & Inotropes

Drug	Alpha	Beta$_1$	Beta$_2$
Phenylephrine	++++	-	-
Norepinephrine	++++	++	-
Epinephrine	++++	++++	++
Dopamine	++ < 5mcg/kg/min	++++ < 10 mcg/kg/min	+
	+++ > 10mcg/kg/min		
Dobutamine	+	++++	++

Adrenergic receptors:

» Alpha—located in blood vessels

» Beta$_1$— located on the heart

» Beta$_2$— located in the bronchial & vascular smooth muscle

Vasopressors (Used to increase blood pressure):

Dopamine (Inotropin)

» Effect: ↑HR, ↑BP

» Classified as a catecholamine

» Acts on the sympathetic nervous system (SNS)

» Positive inotropic effects

» Monitor closely for extravasation

» Stimulates Beta$_1$ & some Beta$_2$, alpha

» Watch out for tachy arrhythmias & ventricular ectopy

Dosing:

- » 0.5 - 3 mcg/kg/min—dopaminergic receptors

- » 3 - 10 mcg/kg/min—beta effects (+ inotrope)

- » > 10 mcg/kg/min—alpha effects (vasoconstriction)

- » Max. 20 mcg/kg/min

Norepinephrine (Levophed)

- » Effect: ↑ BP

- » Alpha & Beta$_1$

- » Adverse effects: bradycardia, dysrhythmias, HTN, renal artery vasoconstriction

- » Dosing: 0.5 – 30 mcg/min—titrate to effect

- » Monitor closely for extravasation

Epinephrine (Adrenalin)

- » Effect: ↑ BP, ↑HR

- » Alpha, Beta$_1$, some Beta$_2$

- » Adverse effects: tachycardia, dysrhythmias, chest pain

- » Dosing: 2 - 10 mcg/min—titrate to effect

- » Monitor closely for extravasation

- » Causes hyperglycemia

Phenylephrine (Neo-Synephrine)

- » Effect: ↑ BP

- » Pure alpha

- » Adverse effects: reflexive bradycardia, dysrhythmias, HTN, chest pain

- » Dosing: 2 - 10 mcg/kg/min

- » Titrate to effect/BP parameters established

- » Monitor closely for extravasation

Positive Inotropes (Used to improve cardiac output & contractility):

Dobutamine (Dobutrex)

» Effect: ↑ C.O., ↑ HR

» Stimulates beta receptors, Beta$_1$ (some alpha)

» Also used in cardiac surgery & septic shock

» Dosing: 2.5 – 20 mcg/kg/min IV (up to 40 mcg/kg/min)

» Onset 1 - 2 minutes, up to 10 min.

» Plasma half-life 2 min.

» Monitor for: tachycardia, hypertension, ectopy, hypokalemia

Milrinone (Primacor)

» Effect ↑ C.O., ↓PAOP & SVR, no change in HR

» Phosphodiesterase (PDE) inhibitor

» Vasodilatory effects—watch BP!

» Dosing: Bolus 50 mcg/ kg over 10 min.

  * Maintenance: 0.375 – 0.75 mcg/kg/min

» Long half-life!!!!

  * ~ 6 hours

Vasodilators (Used to decrease SVR or resistance):

Nitroprusside (Nipride)

» Antihypertensive of nitrate origin

» Dosing: 0.5 – 8 mcg/kg/min

» Closely monitor for:

  * Hypotension (check BP Q 1 - 2 min until BP is stabilized)

  * Arterial line preferred if titrating

  * Hypoxia (from intrapulmonary shunt)

  * Increased HR (Stimulation of baroreceptors)

  * Thiocyanate poisoning (esp. if given > 72 hrs.), monitor levels

  * Methemoglobinemia (Hgb can get converted)

Cardiac Surgery

Coronary Artery Bypass Graft (CABG)

» Artery harvested from:

  * Saphenous vein (leg)

  * Internal mammary

  * Radial artery

Post-op considerations:

» Longer cardiopulmonary bypass time =

  * Increased risk of bleeding

  * Increased risk of stroke and neurologic injury

Monitor:

» BP (↑ BP = risk for bleeding)

» Pain

» Electrolyte imbalances

» Bleeding

» Post op ischemia

» Dysrhythmias/blocks

  * Atrial fibrillation

» Hypothermia

  * Vasoconstriction

  * Coagulopathies

Teaching after surgery:

» Signs of infection

» Weight gain

» Heart healthy diet

» Activity/Exercise

» Smoking cessation

» Medication adherence

» Sternal precautions

Cardiac Tamponade

» Compression of the heart due to fluid accumulation within the pericardium

» The pericardial space normally contains 20 – 50 ml of pericardial fluid

» Clinical signs/symptoms of cardiac tamponade:

  • **Beck's Triad**:

    ▷ Elevated CVP w/JVD, hypotension, muffled heart sounds

• Sudden drop in chest tube output

• Narrow pulse pressure (SBP – DBP = PP)

  ▷ Normal PP = 40 mm Hg

• Tachycardia

• Electrical alternans

  ▷ Alternating beat variation of amplitude on ECG

• Pulsus paradoxus

  ▷ > 10 mm Hg drop in BP during inspiration

• Pulseless Electrical Activity (PEA)

Treatment of cardiac tamponade:

» Pericardiocentesis

  • Risk: Laceration of coronary artery

» Median re-sternotomy

» Goal: Locate & control source of bleeding

Treatment of atrial fibrillation/atrial flutter

General risk factors for developing afib/aflutter:

» CABG

» Valvular disease

» MI

» Atherosclerosis

» Rheumatic heart disease

» Lung disease

Rates can vary:

» < 100 bpm

» > 100 bpm "Rapid ventricular response"

» Lose atrial kick

» ↓ in CO by up to 20 - 25%

Management of afib/aflutter:

Rate control vs. conversion

» Synchronized cardioversion if new (vs. chronic) & unstable

» Digoxin

» Beta blockers (esmolol, metoprolol)
  * Use cautiously in patients with reduced EF
  * Has negative inotropic effects

» Calcium channel blockers (diltiazem)~~⁄~~
  * Use cautiously in patients with reduced EF
  * Has negative inotropic effects

~~»~~ Amiodarone—safer to use with reduced ejection fraction

» Anticoagulation if sustained in afib

Heart Failure

2 types:

Heart Failure with preserved EF (HFpEF)

» **Diastolic Heart Failure**

» Ejection Fraction (EF) ≥ 50%

» Borderline EF 41 – 49%

» Stiff non-compliant ventricle

» Usually history of hypertension

Heart Failure with reduced EF (HFrEF)

» **Systolic Heart Failure**

» Ejection Fraction ≤ 40%

» aka: "congestive heart failure"

» Acute decompensated HF

» Know this one for the exam!

Ventricular failure—left vs. right side

Left sided failure—blood backs up to the lungs

» Tachypnea

» Tachycardia

» S_3 heart sound

» Mitral regurgitation

» Displaced point of maximal impulse (PMI)

» Crackles

» Cough, frothy sputum

» ↑ PA pressures

» ↑ PAOP

» ↓CO/CI

Right sided failure—blood backs up to the venous periphery

» JVD

» Hepatojugular reflux

» Peripheral edema

» Hepatomegaly

» Anorexia, N/V

» Ascites

» Tricuspid regurgitation

» ↑CVP/RAP

» ↑Liver enzymes

Assessment in heart failure:

PMI (Point of maximum impulse)

» Normally palpated at the 5th ICS, MCL

Causes of PMI shifting:

» Left ventricular hypertrophy

» Heart failure

» Right pneumothorax

» Right pleural effusion

Measuring JVD

» Supine position, HOB 30°

» Turn head slightly to left—note: the right jugular is aligned directly with the right atrium

» Observe for pulsations

» Note highest point

» Measure distance between the pulsation and sternal angle

» 4 cm above sternal angle is normal

Heart failure (HFrEF)

HFrEF - Reduced EF Systolic Heart Failure

» Damage to myofibrils

» ↑ preload & afterload

» Elevated BNP Levels

  • Hormone secreted by ventricles in response to stretch

General medical management

All aimed at blocking the sympathetic nervous system (SNS) and renin angiotensin aldosterone system (RAAS)

» ACE inhibitor OR angiotensin receptor blocker (ARB)

» Beta-blocker OR alpha/beta blocker (i.e. Carvedilol)

» Aldosterone antagonist (i.e. spironolactone)

» Hydralazine (afterload reducer)

» Vasodilators (nitrates)

» Diuretics (usually loop)

» Cardiac glycosides (i.e. digoxin)

Acute decompensated heart failure

» Dobutamine or Milrinone infusions

  • Improve contractility, decrease afterload

» Diuretics

  • Decrease preload

» Nesiritide (Natrecor)

  • Sometimes used in acute decompensated HF without cardiogenic shock

* Potent vasodilator
* Dilates arteries and ↓SVR, ↓PAOP, ↑ C.O.
* Inhibits the renin-angiotensin-aldosterone system

* Dosing: bolus 2 mcg/kg over 1 minute
* Maintenance: 0.01 mcg/kg/min
* Short half-life (~18 minutes)
* Monitor for hypotension

Long term heart failure options

» Biventricular pacing if the patient has a BBB

» Cardiac assist devices (LVAD, RVAD or BiVAD)

» Cardiac transplant

» + Inotropes (i.e. Dobutamine or Milrinone)—can be used palliative

Ventricular Assist Device (VADS)

» Left (LVAD), right (RVAD) or both (BiVAD)

Short term

» Bridge to transplant

Long term

» Destination therapy LVAD

Cardiac transplantation

» Vagal nerve is severed

» Atropine will not work if bradycardia develops—need to pace!

» Immunosuppression to prevent rejection

» Prevent infection!

Cardiac Resynchronization Therapy

» Biventricular Pacemaker

» Used in heart failure when patient has low EF & BBB

» Bi-ventricular pacing results in shortened QRS duration

Benefits:

* Synchronized ventricular contraction

* Increased EF/C.O.

* Symptom improvement

* Complement medical therapy

* Improve quality of life

* Give hope to those who are suffering with moderate to severe heart failure

* No mortality benefits shown

Heart Failure Diagnostics

» 12 Lead ECG—Assess for ischemia, BBB

» Chest radiograph—assess for fluid overload

» ECHO

» Trans-Esophageal Echo (TEE)—assess heart function and presence of thrombus

» Angiogram indicated if ischemic

Heart Failure Discharge Education

» Medication adherence

» Activity

» Daily weight

» Sodium restricted diet

* *Na^+ & fluid restriction debatable; fluid restrict if hyponatremic, Na^+ restrict if pulmonary congestion

» Smoking (and other health habits—quit smoking, limit alcohol intake, lose weight)

» Prevent infection—flu & pneumococcal vaccines

Hypertrophic Obstructive Cardiomyopathy (HOCM)

Physiologic changes:

» Thickened interventricular septum

» Diastolic dysfunction

» Decreased compliance & aortic outflow obstruction

» May present with sudden cardiac death

» Assessment: S_4, murmur, displaced PMI,

» Treatment: beta blockers and calcium channel blockers

» Goal—prolong diastole & filling time!

» Avoid inotropes!!! (i.e. Digoxin/Dobutamine)

» Surgical options: Percutaneous transluminal septal myocardial ablation (PTSMA)

» Septal Myomectomy—removing septal muscle that is contributing to aortic outflow obstruction

» Implantable Cardioverter Defibrillator (ICD)— prevent sudden cardiac death

Takotsubo Cardiomyopathy

» Also called "Broken Heart Syndrome" or "Stress Induced Cardiomyopathy"

» Result of severe emotional or physical stress

» Possibly the result of a surge in stress hormones (i.e. adrenalin)

» Weakening & ballooning of the left ventricle

» Reversible, happens almost exclusively in women

» Often resolves within one month

Symptoms:

» Chest pain

» SOB

» Can see ST elevations on the 12 Lead ECG

» Coronary cath is often clean

Treatment:

» Standard heart failure meds—ACE
inhibitor or ARB, beta blocker,
loop diuretics, aldosterone
antagonists (spironolactone)

Murmurs & Valve Dysfunction

Murmurs—2 causes:

» Forward flow of blood through
stenotic open valves

» Backward flow through
incompetent closed valves

» Murmurs are high pitched
except murmurs of stenosis

Systolic murmurs

» Pulmonary & aortic sten<u>O</u>sis
are systolic murmurs...

* Murmurs of sten<u>O</u>sis
are auscultated when
valves are <u>O</u>pen!

* The pulmonic & aortic valves
are <u>O</u>pen during systole

* Therefore, they are
systolic murmurs!

» Tricuspid & mitral
regurg/insufficiency are
systolic murmurs...

* Murmurs of insufficiency
are auscultated when
valves are closed!

* The tricuspid & mitral valves
are closed during systole

* Therefore, they are
systolic murmurs!

» Auscultate on and between
S_1 and S_2 (during systole)

» S_1 - murmur - S_2

Diastolic murmurs

» Tricuspid & mitral sten<u>O</u>sis
are diastolic murmurs...

* Murmurs of sten<u>O</u>sis
are auscultated when
valves are <u>O</u>pen!

- The tricuspid & mitral valves are Open during diastole

- Therefore, they are diastolic murmurs!

» Pulmonary & aortic regurgitation/insufficiency are diastolic murmurs...

- Murmurs of insufficiency are auscultated when valves are closed!

- The tricuspid & mitral valves are closed during diastole

- Therefore, they are diastolic murmurs

» Auscultate after S_2 (during diastole)

» S_1 - S_2 - murmur

Type of murmur	Systolic or Diastolic?	Location
Mitral Stenosis	Diastolic	5th ICS, MCL
Mitral Regurg	Systolic	5th ICS, MCL
Aortic Stenosis	Systolic	2nd ICS, RSB
Aortic Regurg	Diastolic	2nd ICS, RSB

Valvular Dysfunction

Mitral Insufficiency/Regurgitation

» Systolic murmur

Causes:

» MI

» Ruptured chordae tendineae

» Severe left heart failure

» Left ventricular hypertrophy

» Cardiomyopathy

» Mitral valve prolapse

» Rheumatic fever

Treatment:

» Mitral valve clip (if a candidate)

» Mitral valve replacement

Mitral Stenosis

» Auscultate when the mitral valve is OPEN

» Diastolic murmur

» Signs & symptoms:
   * Pinkish cheeks
   * Pulmonary edema
   * Prone to afib

Treatment:

» Medical management

» Surgical replacement

» Balloon Valvuloplasty (increase diameter/opening of valve)

Aortic Insufficiency/Regurgitation

» Diastolic murmur

» Results in a backflow of blood & reduced diastolic pressure

Causes:

» Chronic hypertension

» Rheumatic fever

» Endocarditis

» Idiopathic—means we don't know why!

Symptoms:

» DeMusset sign—head bobbing

» Brisk carotid upstroke

» Wide pulse pressure
- > 40 mm Hg (high systolic BP; low diastolic BP)

» "Water-hammer" pulse— rapid upstroke & down stroke with a shortened peak

Associated with:

» Marfan's Syndrome

» Ventricular septal defect (VSD)

Aortic Stenosis

» Auscultate when the
aortic valve is <u>O</u>PEN

» Systolic murmur

» Systolic ejection is impeded

» Pressure gradient
between LV & aorta

» 50%, 2-year mortality
if HF develops

Symptoms:

» Heart failure

» SOB

» Activity intolerance

Treatment:

» Valve replacement

» Trans-Catheter Aortic Valve
Replacement (TAVR)

Valvular diagnosis

» Echocardiogram (gold standard)

» Cardiac catheterization (↑LVEDP,
↑atrial pressure, ↑PAOP, ↓CO)

» 12 lead ECG: left atrial &
ventricular hypertrophy

» Chest x-ray: left atrial &
ventricular enlargement,
pulmonary venous congestion

Treatment:

» Treat heart failure if present:

* ACE inhibitor or ARB

* Beta blocker (blunt
the SNS & RAAS)

* Diuretics

* Afterload reduction (hydralazine)

» Valve repair/replacement

Acute Inflammatory Diseases

Myocarditis

» Focal or diffuse inflammation of the myocardium

» Viral or bacterial infection

Clinical signs:

» Fever, chest pain, heart failure, dysrhythmias, sudden cardiac death

» May be accompanied by pericarditis

Treatment:

» Antibiotics (if bacterial)

» + inotropes

» NSAIDs

» ACE inhibitor

» Diuretics

Pericarditis

» Inflammation of the pericardial sac

» Restrictive: effusions into the pericardial sac

» Constrictive: fibrous deposits on the pericardium

Causes:

» Acute MI, post-CABG, connective tissue disease, infection

• Caused from an autoimmune response or viral infection

» Dressler's syndrome:

» 10 - 15% develop this 2 - 7 days after AMI

• 2 - 12 weeks after MI

Symptoms:

» Fever

» Chest pain worse with deep breath, relieved by leaning forward

» Non-specific ST segment changes in the precordial leads

» Diffuse ST segment elevation on 12 lead ECG

Endocarditis

» Infection of the endocardium or valve

» Damaged leaflets

Causes:

» Trauma

» Bacteria

At risk:

» Cardiac surgery, rheumatic heart disease, dental procedures, IV drug abuse (especially tricuspid & pulmonic valve)

Symptoms:

» Stabbing, sharp pain (worse on inspiration)

» SOB, cough

» JVD

» Pulsus paradoxus

» Pericardial friction rub

» ST elevations

» Narrow pulse pressure

» Elevated WBC, ESR

Endocarditis common organisms:

» Streptococcus

» Staphylococcus

» Gram negative bacilli

» Fungus (i.e. candida)

» Administer appropriate antibiotics

Assessment findings with inflammatory diseases:

Pulsus paradoxus

» Decrease in systolic pressure during inspiration; > 10 mm Hg

» Caused by cardiac tamponade, pleural effusion, pericarditis or dehydration

Pulsus alternans

» Finding on arterial waveform showing alternating strong and weak beats

» Indicative of left ventricular systolic impairment

Pericardial Rubs

» Scratching, grating, squeaking leather quality

» Left lower sternal border, leaning forward or lying supine in deep expiration

» High frequency

» 3 sounds are present

  • One systolic—occurs anywhere in systole

  • Two diastolic—occurs w/ ventricular stretch at early and late diastole

» Auscultated in MI, pericarditis, autoimmune, trauma, s/p cardiac surgery, autoimmune diseases

Overall "itis" treatment goals:

» Prevent/relieve symptoms
(lean forward)

» NSAIDs (ASA or indomethacin)

» Treat infection

» Corticosteroids

» Chronic: partial pericardiectomy

   * Window is created allowing
fluids to drain into pleural space

» Constrictive pericarditis:
total pericardiectomy

Cardiac Arrest & Resuscitation

» Early CPR with **minimal**
interruptions

» Compressions of good quality

   * 100 - 120/minute

   * 2 - 2.4 inch depth

» Early defibrillation

» Avoid excessive ventilation

   * 10 breaths/min

» Figure out cause

   * 5 H's, 5 T's

Post-arrest care

» Optimize hemodynamics

   * Avoid hypotension

   * Avoid hypoxemia or hyperoxemia

» Reperfusion

   * Does the patient need to
go to the Cath lab?

   * Obtain 12 Lead ECG

» Targeted Temperature
Management (TTM)

   * 32 - 36°C for 24 hours

   * Recommended for all rhythms
& in-hospital arrest

      ▷ Reason: neuro protection

   * Avoid fever once TTM
protocol is complete

   * See Neurology section
for more info

Types of arrest & treatment strategies:

» **Ventricular Fibrillation**

- **S**hock (if readily available); Repeat Q 2 min.
- **C**PR for 2 min
- **R**hythm check - shock if warranted
- **E**pi 1 mg IV/IO Q 3 - 5 min
- **A**miodorone 300 mg IV/IO; repeat bolus 150 mg IV/IO if still in VF/VT
- **M**edications (other): Lidocaine 1.0 - 1.5 mg/kg IV/IO

» **Torsades de pointes**

- Shift in axis
- Caused by hypomagnesemia, prolonged QT, multiple medications
- Also caused by methadone & some quinolones (cause prolonged QT interval)
- Treatment: magnesium sulfate 1 - 2 grams IV/IO (diluted)
- Magnesium antagonist: calcium chloride

» **PEA (pulseless electrical activity)**

- **P**ump: Start compressions
- **E**pinephrine 1 mg IV/IO Q 3 - 5 min
- **A**ssess causes
- **5 H's:**
  - Hypovolemia
  - Hypoxia
  - Hypo/Hyperkalemia
  - H+ ion (acidosis)
  - Hypothermia
- **5 T's:**
  - Thrombus:
    - MI
    - PE
  - Tension pneumothorax
  - Tamponade
  - Toxicology (drug OD)

» **Asystole**

- No cardiac output
- **P**ump (Same as PEA)
- **E**pinephrine 1 mg IV/IO Q 3 - 5 min
- **A**ssess differential diagnosis
- Consider termination if Capnography < 10 mm Hg after 20 min

» **Capnography during resuscitation**

- Used as a marker of perfusion
- Normal PEtCO$_2$ 35 - 45 mm HG
- Minimum goal > 10 mm HG
- If less than 10, improve quality of compressions
- If rapid increase in PEtCO$_2$, may be a sign of ROSC

* If consistently < 10 mm Hg in the setting of adequate compressions, discuss termination of resuscitation efforts

» Tachycardia—Narrow complex

* Stable vs. unstable

* Unstable: Prepare for cardioversion!

* Stable? Narrow & regular complex?

  ▷ **V**agal maneuvers

  ▷ **A**denosine

    ▷ Dosed: 6 mg, 12 mg, 12 mg by RAPID IVP

    ▷ Used in SVT

  ▷ Depresses AV node conduction

  ▷ Instruct patient prior to administration

  ▷ **D**iltiazem IV

» Tachycardia—Wide complex

* QRS > 0.12 sec.; consult an expert

* Amiodarone 150 mg IV over 10 min.

* Can also use Lidocaine for monomorphic wide complex tachycardia

* Since 2010 AHA ACLS guidelines:

  ▷ Adenosine 6 mg IV, may repeat

Conduction issues

Long QT syndrome (LQTS)

» Delayed repolarization can cause Torsade de Pointes (polymorphic ventricular tachycardia)

» Present with fainting or sudden cardiac death

» Prolonged QT, QTc > 450 ms

» Can also result from malnutrition due to K^+ & Mg^{++} deficiencies

Treatment:

» Genetic testing

» Electrolyte supplements

» Beta blockers

» Antidysrhythmic based on cause of LQTS

» Implantable cardioverter defibrillator (ICD)

Brugada Syndrome

» Genetic cause of sudden cardiac death

» Sodium channelopathy

Symptoms:

» Fainting, irregular heart beats

» Coved or saddle-back ST elevations in leads $V_1 - V_3$

» Often have a right BBB

» Long PR interval

» May have short QT interval; < 360 ms

» Structural right ventricle pathology

Treatment:

» Implantable cardioverter defibrillator (ICD)

» Possibly quinidine

Antidysrhythmic Medications:

» Procainamide (Pronestyl)—Class 1A, prolongs repolarization

- Used for atrial dysrhythmias & ventricular tachycardia
- Monitor QTc closely!

» Lidocaine (Xylocaine)— Class 1B, shortens action potential duration

- Used for ventricular dysrhythmias
- Watch for neuro-toxicity

» Flecainide (Tambocor)—Class 1C, blocks Na^+ channels

- Used for ventricular dysrhythmias

» Esmolol (Brevibloc)— Class II, decreases HR & SA node automaticity

- Beta blocker used for atrial dysrhythmias & SVT

» Amiodarone (Cordarone)— Class III, blocks K^+ channels & slows conduction

- Atrial & ventricular dysrhythmias

» Verapamil (Calan)—Class IV, calcium channel antagonist

- Atrial tachycardia & atrial flutter

» Diltiazem (Cardizem)—Class IV, calcium channel antagonist

* Atrial tachycardia & atrial flutter

» Digoxin (Lanoxin)—slows AV node conduction, depressed SA node

* Atrial fibrillation, atrial flutter & SVT

» Adenosine (Adenocard)— slows AV node conduction, depressed SA node

* Atrial flutter & SVT

» Ibutilide (Corvert)

* Class II, Cardio-conversion of atrial flutter & atrial fibrillation

* Better for atrial flutter

Wolfe-Parkinson-White (WPW)

» Pre-excitation

» Abnormal conduction pathway between the atria & ventricles

» Accessory pathways conduct faster than the AV node

» Short PR interval < 0.12

» Delta wave—slurred upstroke in the QRS

Treatment:

» Ablation of the accessory pathway

» Antiarrhythmic medications slow conduction

* Beta blockers often used

Pacemaker Review

» Permanent or temporary

» Indications: symptomatic bradycardia, 2nd degree AV block (Mobitz II), third degree AV block (complete heart block)

» Patients admitted with "Syncope" will require f/u electrophysiology study

» Modes: synchronous (demand) or asynchronous (non-demand)

* Avoid using asynchronous mode

- Will pace regardless of patient's intrinsic rhythm

- Potential issue: R on T, causing lethal dysrhythmias

  » Transcutaneous, transvenous, epicardial

Temporary—Transcutaneous Pacing

» Pad placement: Anterior—posterior or anterior—lateral

» Settings

» Demand (synchronous)

» Fixed (asynchronous)

» More energy required vs. transvenous (start @ 50 mA & increase until capture)

- Need to pace through skin, bone, muscle

Temporary—Transvenous/Epicardial

Pacemaker codes: Example—VVI, AAI, DDD

» First letter: Chamber paced (A, V or D)

» Second letter: Chamber sensed (A, V or D)

» Third letter: Response to sensing

- I—Inhibits pacing if QRS is sensed, demand

- D—Triggers & inhibits pacing
- O—None
- Typically, we want the response to pacing set in either I or D
- This means if the patient has their own intrinsic rhythm, the pacemaker will sense it and not compete with the patient

Examples:

- VVI – V: ventricle is paced, V: ventricle is sensed, I: pacing will be inhibited if the pacemaker senses intrinsic conduction

- DDD – D: atria & ventricle are paced, D: atria & ventricle are sensed, D: pacing will be inhibited if the pacemaker senses intrinsic conduction

Failure to capture:

» Electrical stimulus delivered (pacing spike), but no electrical capture (wide QRS)

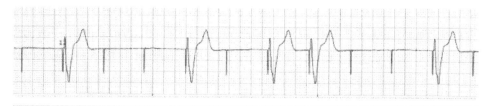

Causes:

» Improper position of wire or pads

» Low voltage

» Battery failure

» Inadequate/loose connection

» Fibrosis of catheter tip

Trouble-shooting:

» Check connections

» Increase mA (energy)

» Assess pH, electrolyte imbalances, ischemia & drug toxicity

* May require much higher mA to capture

Failure to pace:

» No pacing stimulus is delivered

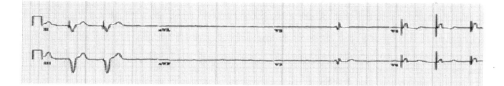

Causes:

» Battery failure

» Loose connections

» Lead dislodgement

» Improper settings

Troubleshooting:

» Assess leads & connections

» Change battery

» Assess thresholds

» Prepare for transcutaneous pacing (TCP)

» Assess labs

Failure to sense:

» Under-sensing: the pacemaker does not recognize intrinsic beats

» Over-sensing: the pacemaker thinks that either p waves or t waves are ventricular depolarization and does not pace

   • Dangerous, because patient can experience R on T phenomenon

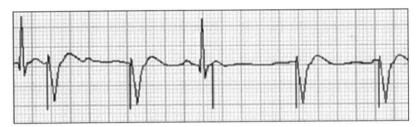

Causes:

» Improper sensitivity settings

» Position of the lead

Troubleshooting:

» Assess thresholds

Magnet Operation with Permanent Pacemakers & ICDs

» A magnet placed over a pacemaker causes asynchronous pacing at a designated "magnet" rate

  * Does NOT turn off the pacemaker...a common misconception!!!

» Over an ICD, a magnet inhibits defibrillation

» A magnet might be used in surgery if cautery is used or if a defibrillator is mis-firing

» Terminates pacemaker mediated tachycardia

Cardiac Trauma

Penetrating trauma, common injury to:

» Chambers of the heart

» Right ventricle

» Pericardium

» Great vessels/coronary arteries

» Risk of infection

» Surgical emergency

Blunt trauma, common causes:

» MVC/steering wheel to chest

» Direct blow to chest

» Fall

» Stunned or contused myocardium

» Ventricular rupture

» Acceleration/deceleration injury: vessel damage

» Direct transfer mechanics

Blunt Cardiac Injury

» Formerly called "cardiac contusion"

» Right atrium & ventricle most at risk

Monitor for:

» Dysrhythmias

» Heart block/right BBB

Medical management:

» Prevent complications

» Heart failure

» Antidysrhythmics

» Temporary pacing

Diagnosis:

» Echo, 12 Lead ECG, CXR, CT Scan, MRI, Trans Esophageal Echo (TEE)

» Cardiac enzymes

» Other labs: Coags, electrolytes, CBC

Hypertension

Category	SBP	DBP
Optimal	< 120	< 80
Pre-hypertension	120 - 139	80 - 89
Stage 1 HTN	140 - 159	90 - 99
Stage 2 HTN	> 160	≥ 100

Source: AHA Guidelines

Long term BP Goals:

≥ 60 years of age:

» SBP < 150 mm Hg and
DBP < 90 mm Hg

≤ 60 years of age:

» SBP < 140 mm Hg and
DBP < 90 mm Hg

4 types of medications recommended:

» Thiazide diuretic

» Calcium channel blocker

» ACE inhibitor

» Angiotensin receptor
blocker (ARB)

Hypertensive Crisis

Acute BP elevation associated with organ damage

» Kidney: decreased blood flow,
hematuria, proteinuria

» Brain: hypertensive
encephalopathy

» Heart: LVH, LVF, MI

» Eyes: retinal hemorrhages

» Vascular system: vessel damage

Treatment:

» BP in both arms (r/o aneurysm
or steal syndrome)

» Consider 12 Lead ECG

» Decrease BP by 25% in 1 - 2 hrs

» IV anti-hypertensives
(vasodilators, diuretics, etc.)

* Nitroprusside
* Labetalol
* Esmolol
* Nicardipine

Aneurysms

Definition: permanent localized dilation of aorta 1.5 times diameter

» Patients will often describe "ripping" chest pain radiating to the back

» > 6 cm associated with increased risk of rupture

Types:

» Thoracic (TAA)

» Abdominal (AAA)

» Aortic dissection

» Rupture

» Leaking

Thoracic Aneurysm

» At risk: HTN, smoking

» Dilatation of the aorta > 50% of its normal diameter

» Goal: Prevent rupture or dissection

Treatment:

» BP control/HR reduction

» Surgical repair

BP reducing medications:

» Esmolol (Brevibloc) - short acting, beta blocker

  • Initial dose: 250 - 500 mcg/kg IV over 1 min

  • Maintenance dose: 50 – 200 mcg/kg/min IV infusion

» Labetalol (Trandate)- Blocks alpha, B_1 & B_2 receptors

  • Initial dose: 20 mg IV over 2 min

  • Follow with 20 - 80 mg IV q 10 – 15 min until BP is controlled

- Maintenance dose: 2 mg/min IV continuous infusion; titrate up to 5 - 20 mg/min; not to exceed total dose of 300 mg

» Metoprolol

- Dose: 5 mg IV every 2 min, up to 3 times

» Nitroprusside (Nipride)

- Arteriolar & venous vasodilation

- Starting dose: 0.3 mcg/kg/min; maximum dose 10 mcg/kg/min IV

- Assess thiocyanate levels after 24 – 48 hours for toxicity

» Nicardipine (Cardene)

- Calcium channel blocker

- 5 – 15 mg/hour; minimally titrated

- Direct arterial vasodilator

Abdominal Aneurysm

» Pulsation in the abdomen

» Control HTN

» Surgical repair

Signs of rupture:

» Unrelenting back pain

» Hypotension

» Tachycardia

» Shock

Post-Op Aneurysm Repair

» BP control

» Pain management

» Wean from ventilator

» Closely monitor urine output

» Monitor BUN & creatinine (possible ischemia d/t aortic cross-clamp)

» Monitor for bleeding

Aortic Dissection

» Hypertension is a risk factor

» Signs: BP difference of 25 mm Hg or greater between left & right arm

Ascending aorta (Type A)

» At risk for aortic insufficiency

» Diastolic murmur

» Widened pulse pressure

» Bounding pulse

Descending aorta or aortic arch (Type B)

» Often associated with atherosclerosis

» Intermittent or constant chest pain radiating to back

  • Dull pain between shoulders

Medical management

» If dissected, administer vasodilators to keep BP controlled

» Endovascular stenting

» Surgical repair considered when > 6 cm in diameter

Peripheral Arterial Disease

Lower extremity PAD

» 60% have CAD

» Atherosclerosis

» Claudication—can be intermittent with exercise

Risk factors:

» Smoking, DM, Dyslipidemia, HTN, age > 70

» Limb ischemia

Monitor the 7 "P's":

» Pain

» Pallor

» Paresthesia

» Paralysis

» Pulseless

» Poor temperature

» Poor healing

Ankle/Brachial Index (ABI)

» Arm pressure - SBP from brachial artery

» Ankle pressure - SBP from posterior tibial & dorsalis pedis arteries

» Divide ankle pressure by arm

» ABI Value > 0.9 Normal

» < 0.4 severe obstruction

Diagnostics/Treatment

» Doppler studies

» Arteriography

Management:

Goal is to improve perfusion!

» Anticoagulation

  • Antiplatelet agents

  • Thrombolytic agents

» Vasodilators

» Angioplasty

» Stents

» Surgery—bypass

» Amputation

Deep Venous Thrombosis (DVT)

» May have pain and/or swelling in affected extremity

» + Homans' sign
  • Pain in calf with abrupt dorsiflexion of the foot while the knee is flexed at 90°
  • Not a diagnostic indicator

» If shortness of breath develops, consider pulmonary embolism

» Anticoagulation usually with heparin short term, Coumadin long term

» Consider IVC filter if lower extremity DVT

You can do it!

Cardiac Medications

Class	Examples	Indications	Effects	Monitor	Watch out!
ACE Inhibitors	"prils" Class I: Captopril Class II: Enalapril (Vasotec), Ramipril (Altace) Benazepril (Lotensin) Class III: Lisinopril	-CHF/Systolic failure -AMI (EF < 40%) -Anterior wall MI -HTN -Diabetic renal nephropathy	- Vasodilation -↓ preload & afterload -Prevention of myocardial remodeling -Reduce progress of diabetic nephropathy	BP K+ levels	Hypotension Cough Hyperkalemia Angioedema Renal function
Beta Blockers	"olols" **Cardio-selective (blocks B1):** Bisoprolol, Metoprolol SR, Atenolol, Esmolol (IV), Acebutolol, Nebivolol (Bystolic) **Alpha & Beta Blocking:** Labetalol, Carvedilol (Coreg) **Non-selective (blocks B$_1$ & B$_2$):** Propranolol (Inderal), Timolol, Nadolol (Corgard), Sotalol	-HTN -Secondary prevention of MI -Cardiac arrhythmias -Angina -Afib -CHF/Systolic failure	-↓ HR, BP -Negative inotrope, however, decreases myocardial workload -Decreases preload -block endogenous epi & norepi; "stress catecholamine" -Reduces morbidity & mortality in HF	HR BP AV Blocks Heart failure	Bradycardia Hypotension Signs of shock Bronchospasm; Avoid in asthma! Heart block Avoid with cocaine use **Overdose reversal:** Glucagon
Angiotensin II Receptor Blockers (ARBs)	"sartans" Valsartan, Losartan, Candesartan, Olmesartan, Telmisartan	-HTN -CHF/Systolic failure -Diabetic renal nephropathy -Intolerance of ACE Inhibitors	-Vasodilation -Decreases preload & afterload -Reduces secretion of vasopressin	BP K+ levels	Dizziness Headache Hyperkalemia Caution: MI

				K+ levels	Hyperkalemia—especially when used with ACE Inhibitors or ARBs
Aldosterone Blockers	Spironolactone (Aldactone), Eplerenone (Inspra)	Adjunctive therapy in heart failure	-Diuresis -Blocks Na+ reabsorption -Decreases preload & afterload -In combo with other diuretics, reduces cardiac workload -K+ sparing diuretic	K+ levels	Hyperkalemia—especially when used with ACE Inhibitors or ARBs
Calcium Channel Blockers (CCBs)	"pines" **Benzothiazepine class:** Diltiazem (Cardizem) **Phenylalkylamine class:** Verapamil (Calan) **Dihydropyridines:** (little effect on contractility) Amlodipine, nimodipine, nicardipine (IV), Nifedipine, Felodipine	-HTN -Reduce HR -SVT -Afib/flutter -Angina—Prinzmetal's (vasospasm) -Hypertrophic CM -Prevent cerebral artery vasospasm (nimodipine)	-Arterial vasodilation, ↓ SVR -Reduce the force of myocardial contraction -Negative chronotrope -Negative inotrope	HR BP	Heart block Bradycardia Reflexive tachycardia Caution when used with BB **Overdose:** Calcium Chloride & Atropine
Nitrates	Nitroglycerin Isosorbide dinitrate (Isordil), Isosorbide mononitrate (Imdur)	-Angina -Heart failure	-Vasodilation -Venodilation	Low BP Headaches	Hypotension
Hydrazinophthalazine	Hydralazine *Usually prescribed in combo with a BB & diuretic	-Heart failure -HTN	-Vasodilator → SVR & PVR	BP Headaches	Reflexive tachycardia MI/angina

Definitions:
Inotrope—has an effect on contractility, positive inotrope improves contractility, negative inotrope decreases contractility.
Chronotrope—has an effect on heart rate, positive chronotrope increases the heart rate, negative chronotrope decreases the heart rate.

Hemodynamic Review

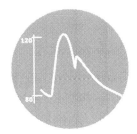

Responsible for:

- Central venous pressure monitoring
- Invasive hemodynamic monitoring
- Intra-Aortic Balloon Pump (IABP)
- Monitor hemodynamic status and recognize signs and symptoms of hemodynamic instability
- SvO_2 monitoring

Hemodynamic Concepts

Cardiac output (C.O.):

- Amount of blood ejected by the ventricles per minute
- C.O. = Heart rate (HR) x Stroke volume (SV)
  - ▷ Normal C.O. = 4 - 8 L/min
  - ▷ Normal cardiac index (C.I.) = 2.5 – 4.0 L/min^2
- Cardiac index = C.O. divided by body surface area (BSA)

» Can be measured by:

- Pulmonary artery catheter
- Echocardiogram
- Indirectly via functional hemodynamics
- Non-invasive methods (ultrasound, Bioreactance technology)

» C.O. may be normal when the patient is tachycardic with lower SV

- In low cardiac output states, compensate with tachycardia

» Stroke volume (SV):

- Normal is 50 - 100 mL/beat
- Normal stroke volume index (SVI) = 35 – 60 mL/beat/m^2
- The amount of blood ejected with each beat

» SV = end diastolic volume (EDV) minus end systolic volume (ESV)

- Typical EDV = 120 ml
  - ▷ Amount of blood in the heart at the end of diastole
- Typical ESV = 50 ml
  - ▷ Amount of blood in the ventricles at the end of ejection/systole

» Three measures contribute to SV:

- Preload
  - ▷ Myocardial fiber length at the end of diastole
- Afterload
  - ▷ Resistance the heart has to eject against during systole
- Contractility
  - ▷ Strength of myofibril contraction

Preload

» Defined as the stretching of cardiac myocytes prior to ejection

» Volume concept, measured as pressure

» End diastole

* Volume of blood filling the ventricle during diastole

» Indirectly measured on the <u>right side</u> of the heart:

* Right Atrial Pressure (RAP)

* Central Venous Pressure (CVP)

* Normal 2 – 6 mm Hg

» Indirectly measured on the <u>left side</u> of the heart:

* Pulmonary Artery Occlusive Pressure (PAOP)

* Normal 8 – 12 mm Hg

* Reflective of left atrial pressure

» Conditions causing an increase in preload:

* Heart failure

* Hypervolemia

* Cardiogenic shock

* RV failure ($\uparrow$CVP)

* Ventricular septal defect (VSD)

* Pulmonary hypertension ($\uparrow$CVP)

* Tricuspid stenosis ($\uparrow$CVP)

* Mitral stenosis ($\uparrow$PAOP)

* Pericardial tamponade ($\uparrow$CVP and $\uparrow$PAOP)

* Increasing PEEP on ventilator

▷ Can also decrease venous return

* IV fluids (at least that's usually the goal)

» Conditions causing a decrease in preload:

* Hypovolemia

* Bleeding

* Veno/vasodilation

* Decreased venous return

* Administration of morphine, NTG, beta blockers or diuretics

Afterload (Systemic Vascular Resistance)

» Defined as the pressure or resistance the ventricles must overcome to eject

» Pulmonary vascular resistance (PVR)

* Normal 90 - 250 dynes/sec/cm^{-5}

» Systemic vascular resistance (SVR)

  * Normal 900 - 1400 dynes/sec/cm^{-5}

  * Formula = MAP – CVP(80) ÷ C.O.

» Conditions causing an increase in afterload:

  * Cardiogenic shock

  * Hypovolemic shock

  * Bleeding

  * Heart failure

  * Cardiac tamponade

  * Use of vasopressors (i.e. epinephrine, norepinephrine)

  * Think **vasoconstriction!**

» Conditions causing a decrease in afterload:

  * Septic shock (warm stage)

  * Anaphylactic shock

  * Spinal/neurogenic shock

  * Insulin shock

  * Vasodilators (i.e. Nitroglycerin, Nipride)

  * Think **vasodilation!**

Contractility

» Force of ventricular ejection

» Difficult to measure

» Influenced by changes in preload & afterload

» "Inotrope" +/-

  * + inotropes will increase contractility (i.e. Dobutamine, Milrinone, digoxin)

  * – inotropes will decrease contractility (i.e. beta blockers)

» Other factors decreasing contractility:

  * STEMI

  * Sepsis

  * Inadequate stretch

  * ↑ Resistance (increased SVR/afterload)

  * ↑ H^+ (acidosis)

  * ↑ CO_2

  * ↓O_2 Supply

SvO_2

» True mixed venous O_2 saturation

» Measures relationship between oxygen delivery & consumption

» Normal oxygen extraction ratio (O_2ER) = 25 – 30%

» In other words, we normally extract 25 – 30% of oxygen to the tissues & 70 – 75% comes back to the heart and is measured via SvO_2 or $ScvO_2$

» Normal SvO_2 60 – 75%

- Measured with a pulmonary artery catheter

- $ScvO_2$ 70% - 85%

- Surrogate of mixed venous —central venous

- Runs about 5 – 8% higher than SvO_2

- If you cannot continuously monitor:

- Draw sample from distal tip of CVC/PICC (thorax) that is positioned in the superior vena cava

If SvO_2 or $ScvO_2$ is low, first ask yourself—is a delivery or consumption problem?

» DO_2 (O_2 delivery) is affected by 3 physiologic parameters:

- "The Pump"—Is the cardiac output adequate? Does the patient need fluid or +inotrope?

- "The Lungs"—Is the oxygenation adequate? Excessive metabolic demands?

- "The Hemoglobin"—Is there adequate O_2 carrying capacity?

» VO_2 (O_2 consumption) is increased by:

- Increased work of breathing

- Shivering

- Fever

- Infection

- Agitation

- Turning/mobility

- Nursing care

The Pulmonary Artery Catheter (PAC)

a.k.a. "Swan-Ganz" catheter

Contraindications to PA catheter insertion:

» Tricuspid or pulmonic prosthetic valve

» Right heart mass (thrombus or tumor)

» Tricuspid or pulmonic valve endocarditis

» Left BBB

Direct measurements from PAC:

» Right atrial pressure (RAP/CVP)

» Pulmonary artery pressures (PAS/PAD)

» Pulmonary artery occlusive pressure (PAOP)

» C.O.

» SvO_2

Calculated measurements:

» SV/SVI

» C.I.

» SVR

» PVR

» DO_2

Guidelines for PAC use:

» Level at phlebostatic axis

  • 4th ICS & ½ AP diameter (level of left atrium)

  • Eliminates effects of hydrostatic forces on the observed hemodynamic

  • Ensure air-fluid interface of the transducer is leveled before zeroing and/or obtaining pressure readings

» 0 - 60° HOB Elevation

» Dynamic response testing (a.k.a square wave test)

  • Fast flush—should see 1 - 3 oscillatory waves following flush

  • Optimal test ensures the line is reliable

» Over-damped waveform

  • Sluggish, artificially rounded & blunted appearance

  • SBP erroneously low; DBP erroneously high

  • Causes: large air bubbles in system, compliant tubing, loose/open connections, and low fluid level in flush bag

» Under-damped waveform

  • Over responsive, exaggerated, artificially spiked waveform

  • SBP erroneously high; DBP erroneously low

  • Causes: small air bubbles, excessive tubing length, defective transducer

Rules for measuring HD waveforms:

» Measure at end-expiration

» Interpret the CVP & PAOP at the mean of the a – c wave

RAP/CVP waveform consists of:

» a wave—upstroke of atrial systole

» c wave—often not visible; represents valve closure

» v wave—atrial diastole when tricuspid valve is closed

* Read the avg. of the "a" & "c" wave <u>or</u>

» Z-point method

* To do this: record the ECG strip with the CVP or PAOP

* Measure where the end of QRS complex intersects with the CVP or PAOP

* This gets you pretty close to the mean a/c wave

Pulmonary artery pressure (PAP)

» Normal PA pressure = 25/10 mm Hg

» Causes of elevated systolic (PAS):

* Pulmonary embolism
* COPD
* ARDS

* Hypoxia
* Pulmonary HTN

» Causes of elevated diastolic (PAD):

* Left ventricular failure
* Mitral valve dysfunction
* Cardiac tamponade

PA diastolic (PAD) is reflective of LVEDP except with:

» Mitral valve dysfunction

» Pulmonary HTN

» Right BBB

» Aortic insufficiency

» Pulmonic insufficiency

» Decreased LV compliance

PAOP "Wedge" pressure

» Normal 8 - 12 mm Hg

» Preload indicator

» Estimates left atrial
filling pressures

» PAOP should be < PAD

» Assumes pressure & volume
are directly proportional

* However, that is only in a
normally compliant ventricle!

* Disproportionate increase
in pressure w/ an increase in
volume in critically ill patients

* Compliance is a change
in pressure for a given
change in volume

Some safety tips for PAOP:

» Inject slowly and stop when
the waveform changes

» Never inject more
than 1.5 ml of air

» Stop inflating the balloon
if resistance is met

» Inflate < 15 seconds

» Allow air to passively exit

» If PA waveform does not
change, this may a sign of:

  ▷ Balloon rupture

  ▷ Tip of PA is in the RV or in
  PA

PAOP waveform consists of:

» a wave = atrial contraction
(after QRS)

» c wave = mitral valve closure

» v wave = Atrial filling
(after T wave)

General PAOP guidelines:

» Elevated in:

  * Mitral stenosis

  * Mitral insufficiency

  * Left ventricular failure

* Fluid/volume overload

* Cardiac tamponade

* Constrictive pericarditis

* High levels of PEEP

Lung zones

» PA Cath tip must be placed in Zone 3

» Signs it's in Zone 1 or 2 (the wrong position):

- Damped paop waveform
- PAOP > PAD
- Absence of a and v waves

Causes of large "V" waves (CVP or PAOP)

» Mitral regurgitation (PAOP)

» Tricuspid regurgitation (CVP)

» Fluid overload (Could be either, primarily PAOP)

» Ventricular septal rupture (CVP)

Shock Hemodynamics

Types of Shock	CO/CI	Preload: CV/PAOP	Afterload: SVR	SvO$_2$	Treatment
Cardiogenic	Decreased	Increased	Increased	Decreased	+ Inotropes afterload pressors
Hypovolemic	Decreased	Decreased	Increased	Decreased	Fluids or blood
Septic Shock	Increased (Warm)	Decreased	Decreased	Decreased	Fluids, Antibiotics, + Inotropes, Pressors
	Decreased (Cold) Late	Increased Late	Increased	Increased Late	
Obstructive (Tamponade)	Decreased	Increased	Increased	Decreased	Pericardiocentesis

Vasopressors & Positive Inotropes: How they affect hemodynamics

Medication	HR	MAP	C.O.	SVR	PAOP
Vasopressors					
Phenylephrine	-	↑↑↑	-	↑↑↑	↑/-
Norepinephrine	↑/-	↑↑↑	↑	↑↑↑	↑/-
Dopamine	↑↑	↑↑	↑↑	↑	↓
Epinephrine	↑↑↑	↑↑↑	↑	↑↑↑	↑/-
Vasopressin	↓/-	↑↑	↓/-	↑↑↑	↑
Positive inotropes					
Dobutamine	↑↑↑	↑/↓	↑↑↑	↓/-	↓
Milrinone	↑	↑/↓	↑↑↑	↓/-	↓
Vasodilators					
Nitroglycerin	-	↓	↑/-	↓	↓↓
Nitroprusside	-	↓↓	↑↑	↓↓	↓↓
Nicardipine		↓↓			
Esmolol	↓	↓	↓/-	↓	↑/-

↑ = little effect, ↑↑ = moderate, ↑↑↑ = major, (-) = not much

Intra-Aortic Balloon Counterpulsation IABC/IABP

» Used in cardiogenic shock & decompensated heart failure

» Balloon inflates during diastole at the dicrotic notch

• Dicrotic notch signifies closure of the aortic valve

• Coronary arteries are perfused during diastole

» Deflates during systole

Contraindications:

» Aortic insufficiency

» Aortic aneurysm

Benefits of IABP:

» Increased coronary artery perfusion

» Increased perfusion to organs

» Increased O_2 supply

» Decreased O_2 demand

» Decreased afterload

Complications of IABP:

» Limb ischemia—due to femoral access

  • Monitor pulses distal to insertion site

» Incorrect timing

» Renal artery occlusion

  • Monitor urine output closely

  • Daily CXR to verify position

» Infection

You can do it!

Endocrine Review

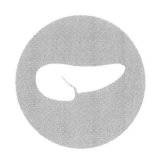

AACN Blueprint for the Endocrine portion for the CCRN® Exam

- Acute hypoglycemia

- Hyperglycemia

- Diabetic ketoacidosis (DKA)

- Hyperglycemic hyperosmolar non-ketotic syndrome (HHNK or HHNS)

- Diabetes insipidus (DI)

- Syndrome of inappropriate secretion of antidiuretic hormone (SIADH)

IV Fluids - Basic Concepts

Physiologic Osmolality

» The measure of solute concentration, defined as the number of osmoles of solute per liter of solution (mOs/L)

» Normal serum osmolality 275 – 295 mOs/L

» **Calculation:** (FYI only)

  • (2 x Na⁺) + (Glucose divided by 18) + (BUN divided by 2.8)

  • OR, if the glucose is normal: The sodium level multiplied by 2, gives a ballpark estimate

Osmolality of IV fluids

Isotonic IV fluids—close to normal serum osmolality

» Normal Saline (308 mOs/L)

» When given, should stay in the vasculature

» Lactated Ringers (273 mOs/L)

Hypertonic Solutions (osmo higher than serum)

» D5 0.2 NS (321 mOs/L)

» D5 ½ NS (406 mOs/L)

» D5LR (525 mOs/L)

» When given, will pull fluid from the cell to the vasculature

» 10% Dextrose (505 mOs/L)

» Hypertonic Saline solutions

  • 2%, 3%, 5%, 23.4% Saline

Hypotonic Solutions (osmo lower than serum)

» 0.45 NS (154 mOs/L)

» When given, will provide cellular hydration

» D_5W (252 mOs/L)—Isotonic in the bag; the body quickly metabolizes the glucose

Acute Hypoglycemia

» Is bad!!! Avoid it!

» Associated with higher mortality!!!

» Defined as serum glucose < 70 mg/dL

» Too much insulin in relation to glucose

» Identify cause; predisposing factors

» Frequent glucose monitoring

» Beta-blockers—Check glucose more frequently

  • Blunt the SNS

  • May not see signs of hypoglycemia

Hypoglycemia causes:

» Too much insulin

» Nausea and/or vomiting

» Interrupted feedings (oral, enteral or parenteral)

» Strenuous exercise or stress (increased metabolic needs)

» Excessive ETOH

» Adrenal insufficiency

» Severe liver disease

» Pregnancy

Hypoglycemia Symptoms:

Cardiovascular (Initial symptoms observed due to activation of the sympathetic nervous system)

» Palpitations

» Tachycardia

» Diaphoresis

» Pallor

» Cool skin

» Piloerection ("goose bumps")

» Irritability

Neurologic symptoms

» Blurred vision

» Slurred speech

» Weakness

» Headache

» Difficulty concentrating

» Confusion

» Fatigue

» Diplopia

» Anxiety

» Tremors

» Staggering gate

Concerns when blood glucose is 20 – 40 mg/dL:

» Seizures

Concerns when blood glucose is < 20 mg/dL:

» Coma

Hypoglycemia Treatment

» If conscious:

  * 4 oz. juice

  * 10 – 15 grams of Carbohydrates

  * Glucose tablets or gel

» If unconscious with IV access:

  * 0.5 to 1 amp of Dextrose 50%

  * Consider 5 - 10% Dextrose in water infusion

» If unconscious without IV access:

  * Glucagon 0.5 – 1 mg IM

» Provide longer acting carbohydrate once stabilized

Metabolic Syndrome

» Estimated 25% of the US population

  * 40% incidence age > 60

» High risk for developing CV disease & DM

Any 2 of the following:

- » Elevated triglycerides > 150 mg/dL

- » Low HDL < 40 in males, < 50 in female

- » Elevated BP: SBP > 130 or DBP > 85

- » Fasting blood glucose > 100 or diagnosed Type 2 DM

- » Waistline > 40 inches men, > 35 inches women

Hyperglycemia & Diabetes Mellitus

- » Fasting BG > 126 mg/dL and $A_1C \geq 6.5\%$

- » Defect in insulin secretion, action of insulin or both

4 Categories of Diabetes Mellitus:

- » **Type 1:** Beta cell destruction resulting in **absolute** insulin **deficiency**

- » **Type 2:** Insulin secretory defect; insulin **resistance** resulting in **relative** insulin deficiency

- » **"Other":** due to other causes; genetic, medication induced

- » **Gestational Diabetes:** due to pregnancy

The pancreas is an endocrine gland:

- » **Alpha cells** produce glucagon

- » **Beta cells** produce insulin

- » **Delta cells** produce somatostatin

HgbA$_1$C

- » Glucose and hemoglobin have a high affinity for each other

- » Estimates the effectiveness of diabetes mellitus therapy

- » Reflective of glucose levels over 3 month period of time

- » Normal value 4 - 5.6% (non-diabetic)

» 6 - 7%: average glucose range 100 - 150 mg/dL

» > 7%: indicative of poorly controlled glucose levels

• Doesn't necessarily mean the patient is non-compliant

• In patients with multiple co-morbid conditions, the goal A_1C may be higher

Limitations of HgbA$_1$C:

» African Americans have greater glycation than other ethnicities

» Unknown if the same cut-off points should be used to diagnose children

» Anemia

Insulin

Action of Insulin

» Drives glucose, water & potassium into cells

» Regular insulin (IV) onset of action: about 5 – 10 min

» Regular insulin (SQ) onset of action: 30 min

• Peak: 2 – 4 hours

• Effects last 5 – 7 hours

Insulin at a glance:

Type	Brand Name	Onset	Peak	Duration
Rapid-acting	Humalog Novolog Apidra	10 - 30 minutes	30 minutes - 3 hours	3 - 5 hours
Short-acting	Regular (R)	30 minutes - 1 hour	2 - 5 hours	Up to 12 hours
Intermediate-acting	NPH (N)	1.5 - 4 hours	4 - 12 hours	Up to 24 hours
Long-acting	Lantus Levemir	0.8 - 4 hours	Minimal peak	Up to 24 hours

Diabetic Ketoacidosis (DKA) & Hyperosmolar Hyperglycemic Syndrome (HHS)

Always look for a cause in DKA & HHS:

» Type 1 DM (DKA)

» Undiagnosed Type 1 DM
(20% of DKA cases)

» Stress

» Illness/Infection

» Trauma

» Surgery

» Non-compliance

» Pancreatitis

» Pregnancy

» Cushing's Syndrome

» Hyperthyroidism

» Diet

» Drugs
  • Thiazide diuretics
  • Glucocorticoids (e.g. prednisone)
  • Diazoxide (hyperstat)
  • Phenytoin
  • Sympathomimetics (e.g. epinephrine, norepinephrine)

Diabetic Ketoacidosis (DKA):

» Lack of insulin leaves too much circulating glucose (drives up the serum osmolality)

» Osmotic diuresis leads to profound water loss (polyuria)

» Leads to glucosuria, dehydration & electrolyte imbalance

Metabolism issues associated with insulin deficiency:

» Accelerated gluconeogenesis

» Glycogenolysis

» Decreased glucose utilization

» Increased lipolysis

» Decreased lipogenesis

» Abundant free fatty acids are converted to **ketone bodies**

Nursing assessment in DKA

» The "3 P's":

* Polyuria (early), oliguria –(late)

* Polydipsia (due to profound water loss)

* Polyphagia (due to ketosis/fat burning)

» Neurologic:

* Headache

* Decreased deep tendon reflexes (DTRs); sluggish & limp

* Visual disturbances

* Hypo/hyperthermia

* Decreased level of consciousness (LOC); may advance to coma

» Cardiovascular:

* Tachycardia

* Decreased central venous pressure (CVP) & pulmonary artery occlusive pressure (because of dehydration)

» Pulmonary:

* Kussmaul's breathing, rapid shallow breathing (blowing off ketones)

* Acetone/fruity odor to breath

» GI:

* Nausea, vomiting

* Abdominal pain

* Weight loss

Laboratory findings in DKA

» Hyperglycemic crisis (BG 300 - 800)

» Metabolic acidosis

* Low pH: if > 7.0 let the patient self-correct, if < 7.0 – consider sodium bicarbonate

* Serum bicarbonate level is often < 20 mEq/L

* Anion gap > 15; often in the 20s

» Elevated serum & urine ketones

» Electrolyte imbalances:

* Increased K^+ (acidosis causes K^+ to shift out of cell)

* Decreased Na^+ & Ca^{++}

Anion gap: Normal < 11 - 12

» Difference between primary measured cations (Na^+ and K^+) and the primary measured anions (Cl^- and HCO_3^-) in serum.

» If the gap is >12; often associated with metabolic acidosis

Here's an easy acronym to remember causes of metabolic acidosis:

M: Methanol

U: Uremia

D: DKA

P: Propylene glycol

I: Isoniazid

L: Lactic acidosis

E: Ethylene glycol

S: Salicylates

Management of Diabetic Ketoacidosis (DKA)

» A fluid deficit should be calculated

* It's often ~ 50 – 100 mL/kg

» Depending on the calculated fluid deficit:

* Administer 1 - 3 liters of IV fluid during the first hour

* Administer 1 L during the second hour

* Administer 1 L during the following 2 hours

* Administer 1 L every 4 hours, depending on the degree of dehydration

» Fluid Management—DKA

* 0.9% Saline or Lactated Ringers (isotonic)

* Add dextrose to the IV Fluids when BG reaches 250 mg/dL (i.e. D5.45)

* Then, 0.45% saline @ 250 - 500 mL/hour (hypotonic)

* Quick tip: Often this last step is skipped if the patient is able to drink water

* Water is hypotonic and will provide cellular hydration.

Insulin Management—DKA

» **Insulin (Regular)**

* Begin infusion at 0.1 units/kg/hour

* Then, insulin infusion goal: decrease glucose SLOWLY!!!

* Do not drop BG by more than 50 - 100 mg/dL per hour

  ▷ Please note: dropping by 100 mg/dL is on the rapid side!

  ▷ Most protocols shoot closer to 50 mg/dL

* Assess blood glucose every 1 - 2 hours until goal is reached

» **Transition to subcutaneous insulin when:**

* The anion gap is corrected

* Ketone body production has ceased (assess serum ketones)

* The glucose is generally less than 200 mg/dL

* Continue to run the insulin infusion for 1 – 2 hours after resuming subcutaneous insulin

  ▷ Prevents patient from going back into DKA

Electrolyte management—DKA

» **Potassium**

* Total body potassium depletion

* Average deficit is 3 – 5 mEq/L

* Serum K^+ is initially elevated in about 22% of cases, normal in about 74% of cases

* Transcellular K^+ shifts with insulin

» **Sodium**

* Dehydration is not reflected in Na^+ levels

* Glucose has a dilutional effect on Na^+

* For every 100 mg/dL increase in glucose, the Na^+ decreases by 1.6 – 2.0 mEq/L

» **Phosphate**

* Depletion is common

* Do not replace unless $PO_4 < 1.0$ mg/dL

* Replacement has little impact on outcome in DKA

» **Magnesium**

* Often depleted

Acidosis—DKA

» K⁺ & pH have an inverse relationship

» For every 0.1 decrease in pH, the serum potassium can increase by 0.6 mEq/L

Quick tip: It's concerning when a patient presents with normal or low potassium levels in the setting of DKA. When insulin & fluids are given there is lots of intracellular shifting and the patient may become severely hypokalemic!

Also, ALWAYS know what the patient's potassium level is prior to administering insulin!

Hyperosmolar Hyperglycemic Syndrome (HHS)

» aka "HHNS", "HHNK", "non-ketotic hyperosmolar hyperglycemia"

» Usually Type 2 DM, can develop in Type I DM as well

- Precipitated by physiologic stress (i.e. trauma, infection, etc.)

- Non-compliance

- Look for a cause!!!

- Review many of the same reasons a patient develops DKA!

Clinical signs of HHS:

» **Absence of ketones**

- Have enough endogenous insulin to prevent ketosis

- Glucose is often > 600, can be >1000 mg/dL

- Polyuria—early sign, then oliguria

  ▷ Urine gets concentrated

▷ Persistent loss of glucose in the urine

- Osmotic diuresis

  ▷ Serum osmo > 330 mOs/L due to dehydration

- Profound **hypovolemia**

- Altered mental status

- Takes days to weeks to develop

HHS—Treatment:

» Volume replacement

* A fluid deficit should be calculated to gauge fluid replacement needs

* Start with isotonic solution (0.9 Saline or LR)

* May need colloids if in hypovolemic shock

* Add dextrose to IV fluids when glucose is lowered to 250 - 300 mg/dL

* Last step: Hypotonic fluids for cellular hydration

  ▷ 0.45% Saline or D_5W (when euvolemic & osmo < 320 mOs/L)

» Insulin (Regular)

* Normalize glucose gradually—will not require as much insulin as DKA

* Monitor serum glucose hourly

* +/- Bolus followed by infusion (mixed opinions about bolus)

Syndrome of Inappropriate Antidiuretic Hormone (SIADH) and Diabetes Insipidus (DI)

Anti-Diuretic Hormone (ADH)

» Purpose of ADH: Maintain fluid balance

» ADH formed in the hypothalamus (brain)

» Released from the posterior pituitary

» Has vasopressor qualities

Syndrome of Inappropriate Anti-Diuretic Hormone (SIADH)

» **Acronym: S**wimming **I**n **ADH**; too much **ADH**

» Water intoxication (kidneys hold onto water & often dilute Na⁺)

Signs:

» **Severe Dilutional Hyponatremia**

* Serum Na⁺ < 120 mEq/L

» Decreased serum osmolality (< 280 mOsm/kg) – d/t dilution

» Urine osmolality > 100 mOsm/ kg H_2O (urine is concentrated)

» Decreased urine output

Causes of SIADH:

» Infection

» Recent surgery (stress)

» Variety of carcinomas/tumors

Complications of SIADH:

» Severe dilutional hyponatremia

» Cerebral edema

» Seizure activity

Treatment of SIADH:

» Safety!!!

» Remedy the problem

» Fluid Restriction

» Hypertonic saline (i.e. 2%, 3%) – temporary

» Assess for fluid overload

* Diuretics (loop diuretics like furosemide)

» Sodium correction:

* Needs to be slow!

* Do not exceed 0.5 mEq/L per hour or 12 mEq/L per day

* If corrected too quickly, can cause demyelination syndrome (permanent neuro damage)

* Do not exceed plasma Na^+ of 130 mEq/L with replacement

Diabetes Insipidus (DI)

» Sip & pis (Sorry, but it's an easy way to remember!)

» Lack of ADH

» Failure of ADH release from the posterior pituitary

» Water loss up to 20 L/day

Common causes (neurogenic most common):

» TBI

» Hypoxic-Ischemic encephalopathy

» Meningitis

» Brain death

» Dilantin

» Tumors

» Can also see nephrogenic causes

DI Symptoms:

» Polyuria

  * Dilute urine (water loss)

  * Urine specific gravity < 1.005 (Dilute)

  * Urine osmolality < 200 mOsm/L (Dilute)

» Extreme polydipsia

» Serum osmolality elevated (> 295 mmol/L)

» Serum Na^+ > 145 mEq/L (d/t H_2O loss)

» Low urine osmolality (50 – 200)

» Low urine specific gravity (< 1.005)

DI Treatment:

» Replace ADH: (IV, IM, SQ, intranasal)

» Desmopressin (DDAVP)

  * IV/SQ: 2 – 4 mcg/day SQ

  * PO: 0.05 mg q 12 hours

  * Intranasal: 10 – 40 mcg/day

» Fluid replacement

» Calculate & replace the free water deficit

» Correct fluid deficit slowly over 2 – 3 days

  * Limits risk of cerebral edema

You can do it!

Gastrointestinal Review

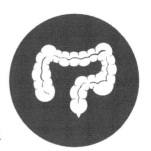

AACN Blueprint for the Gastrointestinal portion of the CCRN© Exam

- Acute abdominal trauma

- Acute GI hemorrhage

- Bowel infarction/obstruction/perforation (i.e. mesenteric ischemia, adhesions)

- Gastroesophageal reflux

- GI surgeries

- Hepatic failure/coma (i.e. portal hypertension, cirrhosis, esophageal varicies, fulminant hepatitis, biliary atresia)

- Malnutrition & malabsorption

- Pancreatitis

Abdominal assessment

Proper order:

» Inspection

» Auscultation

» "Look, listen, feel"

» Percussion

» Palpation—always last!

Small Intestine

» Pyloric sphincter to the cecum

» 18 to 20 feet in length

» Lumen have villi, fingerlike projections to increase surface area

* Aids in digestion

3 segments:

» Duodenum - 10 inches in length

» Jejunum - 8 feet in length

» Ileum - 12 feet

» Major role is digestion & absorption

* Carbohydrates
* Fats
* Protein/Amino acids
* Water
* Electrolytes

Large Intestine

» 5 to 6 feet in length, 2.5 in diameter

» Extends from the ileum to the anus

» Lumen do not have villi like the small intestines

» Responsible for absorption of H_2O, electrolytes & elimination of wastes

Three sections:

» Cecum

» Rectum

» Colon

- Subdivided: Ascending, transverse, descending, sigmoid

Large Intestine Function

» Absorbs 800 – 900 ml fluid

» Bacteria cause formation of gas

» Synthesize vitamin K, thiamine, riboflavin, B12, folic acid, biotin & nicotinic acid

» Main aerobic bacteria is E. coli

Intestinal Infarction

» 20% of the cardiac output goes to the intestines after eating

» Infarction is rare d/t collateral flow

Two main types of infarction:

» Occlusive:

- Embolus or thrombosis to the superior mesenteric artery or major vessel
- Adequate C.O.

» Non-occlusive:

- Associated with decreased C.O. or BP
- At risk: patients with atherosclerosis, heart failure, low C.O. or hypercoagulable state
- Ischemia is secondary to overall low perfusion state

Intestinal Infarction Diagnosis:

» History & clinical presentation

» Rule out other causes

» CT scan—assess for free air (perforation)

» Radiographic angiography

» Assess for embolus or thrombus

» Surgery

- Assess for ischemic or infarcted bowel (more difficult)

Labs:

» Nonspecific

» Leukocytosis

» Follow serial lactate
levels (elevation is a sign
of tissue hypoxia)

» Elevated LDH, amylase

» ABG (metabolic acidosis)

Treatment:

» Adequate resuscitation

Occlusive:

» Angiogram—clot lysis

» Thrombolytic therapy if
present within 8 hours of
onset of symptoms

Non-occlusive:

» Vasodilator therapy to dilate
the mesenteric artery

» Surgery—resect infarcted bowel

» Increase perfusion to gut

• +Inotrope

Bowel obstruction

Causes:

» Adhesions from previous surgery

» Incarcerated hernia

» Tumors

» Ulcers

» Infections

» Abscesses

» Diverticulitis

» Can cause partial or complete obstruction

Signs & symptoms

» Duodenal or proximal small bowel:

- Depends on location & etiology
- **Vomiting
- Crampy, epigastric pain
- Dehydrated

» Distal small bowel or large bowel:

- Vague abdominal pain
- Decreased passing of stool or gas
- Constipation
- Vomiting (late—hours to days after)

Both:

» Decreased PO intake

» Fluid trapped in intestinal loops

» **Early**—bowel sounds are increased, **late**—decreased

Diagnosis:

» Clinical presentation & history

» Abdominal radiograph

- Dilated loops of bowel

» Endoscopy

» CT scan

» Upper GI

» Abdominal ultrasound

Treatment:

» Adequate fluids

» Electrolyte replacement

» Monitor for ileus

- NG tube! (removes air & decompresses stomach)

» Surgery if suspected:

- Adhesions
- Incarcerated hernia
- Diverticuli

» Antibiotics (if indicated)

Gastric perforation

» Rare, can be fatal

» Stomach, duodenum, appendix, colon

» "Rigid" abdomen (guarding)

» Leakage of intestinal content into the peritoneum

» Systemic inflammatory response (SIRS) & infection

  • Tachycardia, tachypnea

  • Fever, leukocytosis & severe abdominal pain

» Elevated Hgb/Hct

  • Hemo-concentrated d/t dehydration

Diagnosis:

» Clinical presentation

» Abdominal films

  • Free air in abdomen

» Exploratory lap—need to go to the OR!

Treatment:

» Surgery

» Adequate volume resuscitation

» Antibiotics

Acute GI Hemorrhage

Upper GI Bleeding:

» Stomach or small intestine

» Ulcers/erosion

» NSAIDS

» Excess acid production

» Stress

» Esophagogastric varicies

» Chronic portal hypertension

» AV Malformations within the intestines

» Mallory-Weiss tear

» Tumor

Symptoms:

» Abdominal pain—
upper quadrants

» Pain worse after eating

» Offenders: ETOH,
aspirin, spicy food

» Vomit blood—bright red
or coffee ground

» Blood in stool (dark)

  • Dumping syndrome—may
    have bright red stool

» > 2 units loss, go into shock

Diagnosis:

» ***Endoscopy

» Active hemorrhage may require
angiography (embolization)

Treatment:

» Maintain optimal hemodynamics

» Crystalloids & transfusions
(if Hgb < 7 mg/dL)

» H$_2$ blockers or PPIs (IV, then PO)

  • Reduces the risk of
    mucosal lining damage

» Vasopressin infusion

  • 0.1 – 0.8 units/min

» Octreotide acetate (Sandostatin)

  • 50 - 150 mcg SQ BID/TID

  • Infusion: 25 - 50 mcg/
    hr x 24 - 48 hrs

Lower GI Bleeding:

» Distal small intestine & colon

» 4 Types:

  • Anatomic

    ▷ Diverticuli—outpouchings
      in intestine

    ▷ Lack of fiber in diet

    ▷ Can become infected &
      bleed

  • Vascular

    ▷ Arteriovenous
      malformations (AVMs)

  • Inflammatory

  • Neoplastic

    ▷ Colon tumors

    ▷ Polyps

Diagnosis & Treatment:

» Colonoscopy

» Barium enema

» Endoscopic or surgical removal

» Severe cases may require embolization or surgery (resection)

» Endoscopic laser, thermal or electrical coagulation

Gastrointestinal Trauma

Blunt "closed" Trauma:

» Motor vehicle collision ("seat belt sign")

» Sports injury

» Risk of bleeding or contusion

Organs at risk:

» Spleen

» Kidney

» Duodenum

» Liver

Penetrating Trauma:

» Stab wounds, gunshot wounds (GSW)

» High risk of bleeding

» Risk of peritonitis

Organs at risk:

» Liver

» Stomach

» Colon

» Spleen

FAST Exam

» **F**ocused **A**ssessment with **S**onography for **T**rauma

» Ultrasound screen for blood around heart & abdominal cavity

Diagnosis:

» CT scan** (gold standard for trauma)

» Identify other organs injured

» Can detect hemorrhage, hematomas, ruptures, lacerations

Treatment:

» IV fluids for resuscitation to maintain hemodynamic stability

» Antibiotics

» Monitor Hgb & Hct

» Surgery if penetrating trauma or active bleeding

» Liver or splenic injury may require arterial embolization

Intra-Abdominal Compartment Syndrome (IACS)

» Increased intra-abdominal pressure from 3rd spacing of fluids

» Associated with fluid resuscitation

» Inflammation

» Capillary leak

Who's at risk?

» Up to 30% of trauma patients

» Over 35% of major abdominal surgery

» Up to 8% of critically ill patients

Signs/Symptoms of abdominal hypertension:

» Abdominal distention

» Decreased urine output

» Intra-abdominal pressure (IAP) > 25 mm Hg

• Normal bladder pressure is 5 – 10 mm Hg

» Abdominal perfusion pressure:

» MAP minus bladder
pressure (IAP)

  * > 60 mm Hg (ideal)

» Respiratory Compromise:

  * Shortness of breath,
    increased respiratory rate

* Increased airway pressure
  (on ventilator)

* Difficult ventilation

» Hemodynamic effects:

  * Decreased venous return
    due to pressure on IVC

  * Decreased C.O.

  * Increased afterload (SVR)

  * Increased preload (CVP/PAOP)

Monitoring/ Treatment:

» Monitor bladder pressure
via bladder catheter

» If IAP > 25 mm Hg –
indication of IACS

» Decompressive laparotomy;
abdomen is left open

» Monitor for organ ischemia

» Follow lactate levels

Hepatic failure

» 75 - 90% of hepatocytes lost
before failure occurs

Functions of the liver:

» Filters toxins

» Filters NH_3 – ammonia

» Synthesize plasma proteins

» Albumin & coagulation factors

Causes of failure:

» Hepatitis

» Fatty liver

» ETOH

» Starvation

» Obesity

» Diabetes

» Advanced cirrhosis

» Hepatic tumors

» Fulminant

» Viral

» Toxin induced
(acetaminophen, ecstasy)

» Ischemia (shock, MODS)

Advanced Cirrhosis

» Hepatic parenchymal
cells destroyed, replaced
with fibrotic tissue

» Constriction of blood flow
leads to portal hypertension

» High risk of developing
liver carcinoma

Physical symptoms:

» Atrophied muscles

» Splenomegaly

» Distended abdomen (ascites)

» Tissue paper thin skin

» Hemorrhoids

» Jaundice

» Lower extremity edema

» Spider angiomas

Labs: (know these!)

» ↓ Albumin, protein

» ↓ Platelet count, fibrinogen

» ↓ Na^+, K^+, Mg^{++}, Ca^{++}, glucose

» ↑ RBCs, ↑/↓ WBCs

» ↑ Hepatic Transaminases

» ↑ AST, ALT, LDH,
alkaline phosphatase

» ↑ AST/ALT ratio > 1 =
chronic failure

» ↑ PTT/PT/INR

» ↑ Lactate

» ↑ Bilirubin

» ↑ Ammonia

» ↑ Aldosterone & ADH

• Contribute to fluid retention

Clinical Presentation:

» Hypotension

» GI Bleed

» Weight loss

» Poor appetite

» Ascites

  • Hydrostatic pressure pushes
    fluid into abdominal space

» Shortness of breath

  • Pressure from ascites
    push on diaphragm

» Chronic low albumin level

» Portal HTN

» Poor renal perfusion

» Jaundice (↑ bilirubin)

  • Usually scleral first

Neuro:

» Lethargic

» Slow to respond

» Slurred speech

» Decreased LOC

» Asterixis

  • Flapping hands

» Hepatic encephalopathy

» Cerebral edema

» Increased ICPs

» Seizures

» Coma

Cirrhosis Diagnosis:

» Liver biopsy

» Ultrasound

  • Assess for portal
    hypertension & nodules

Treatment:

» Treat the cause

» Eliminate cause (ETOH)

» Symptom management

» Evaluate for liver transplant

Ascites Management:

» Low Na⁺ diet

» Little evidence to protein restrict

» Fluid restriction

  * 1.5 L/day

» Diuretics

  * Aldosterone antagonists
    (spironolactone)

  * Loop diuretics

» Paracentesis

  * Not first line treatment

  * Issue with re-accumulation

Nursing Care:

» Measure abdominal girth

» Daily weights

» Monitor labs

» Monitor for hepato-
renal syndrome

  * Oliguria

  * Decreased urine Na⁺

  * Increased BUN/Creatinine

» Monitor for bleeding

  * Vitamin K abnormalities

» Monitor for sepsis

  * Translocation of bacteria from
    GI tract to blood stream

» Monitor neuro changes & LOC

» Drug clearance

  * Caution with sedatives
    (especially benzodiazepines)

» If ammonia elevated—
administer lactulose

  * Poorly absorbed sugar

  * Decreases bowel pH

  * Ammonia excreted in stool

» Nutrition

» TPN or tube feeding if
unable to take PO

» Monitor respiratory status

  * Pressure on diaphragm
    from ascites

Esophageal Varices

Clinical Presentation:

» Dilated, engorged sub-mucosal veins in the mid to distal esophagus

» Caused by chronic portal hypertension

» 30% mortality associated with a bleed

» Elevated liver enzymes, bilirubin, coag times (PT/INR)

» Quickly go into hypovolemic, hemorrhagic shock

Treatment:

» Difficult to control bleeding

» Correct coags

» Airway protection

» Hemodynamic support

» Vasopressin infusion

  • 0.2 – 0.8 unit/min

  • Reduces portal pressure

» Achieve hemostasis:

  • Somatostatin

    ▷ Short acting

    ▷ Causes decrease in portal inflow

  • Octreotide

    ▷ Long acting—continue for up to 5 days post bleed

» Endoscopic banded ligation

» Sclerotherapy

  • High incidence of re-bleed

» Beta blockers (propranolol)

» Nitrates

» Transjugular Intrahepatic Portosystemic Shunting (TIPS)

  • Done in Interventional Radiology

  • Blood directed from the portal vein to the hepatic vein to relieve pressure in the portal system

  • Encephalopathy may develop or worsen

  • Higher risk uncontrolled bleeding

Esophageal Balloon

- Minnesota Tube, Blakemore (brands)
- 2 balloons: gastric & esophageal
- Tamponade bleeding area
- Placement verified via x-ray
- Airway protection is an issue
- Consider endotracheal intubation
- Aspiration

- Safety: Scissors always at the bedside
- High incidence of re-bleeding after removal

» Gastric balloon inflation:

- 250 - 500 cc Blakemore
- 450 - 500 cc Minnesota

Pancreatitis

» Pancreas is composed of head, body & tail

» Endocrine gland
- Secretion of insulin
- Secretion of glucagon

» Exocrine gland
- Release digestive enzymes
- 10% of pancreatic enzymes must be present to prevent malabsorption

Pancreatic enzymes

» Pancreatic amylase
- Alpha amylase released in saliva
- Breaks down carbohydrates
- Breaks down raw & cooked starches

» Lipase
- Digest fats
- Bile salts are essential for this!!!

Acute Pancreatitis

» Acute, local inflammation; triggers systemic inflammation

» Enzymatic auto-digestion of the pancreas

» Enzymes are activated prior to release from the pancreas

» Obstruction of the pancreatic duct can lead to activation of digestive enzymes

» 2 most common causes of duct obstruction:
- ETOH
- Gall stones

Clinical Presentation:

» Pain—upper abdomen, radiates to the back

» Tender, distended abdomen

» Bowel sounds decreased or absent

» Nausea, vomiting

» Fever

» Tachycardia

» Hypotension

» Pleural effusions

  * Left sided or bilateral due to inflamed pancreas near left diaphragm

  * Elevated hemi-diaphragm

  * Atelectasis

» Pulmonary infiltrates

  * Monitor for increasing O_2 needs

  * Monitor for ARDS!!!

Necrotizing Pancreatitis—most severe form

» Necrosis of pancreas, peri-pancreatic tissue & fat

» Hemorrhage

» S/S Hypovolemic shock

» Sequestration of fluids in the peritoneum

» Cullen's sign—ecchymosis around umbilicus

» Grey-Turner's—flank ecchymosis

» May appear within 1 - 2 weeks with hemorrhagic pancreatitis

Diagnosis of Acute Pancreatitis:

» Elevation of amylase*** (elevates within 24 hours)

  * Many times over 500

  * Can return to normal within 3 to 5 days after onset

  * Not a marker of severity

  * Elevated urinary amylase

» Elevated lipase

  * Stays elevated longer than amylase

» Hypocalcemia

  * Follow ionized calcium

  * Calcium binds with fatty acids from necrotic fat

- » H/H—may be increased or decreased (especially later)
- » Leukocytosis
- » Hypoxemia
- » Hypoalbuminemia

- » Hyperglycemia
- » Hypokalemia & hypomagnesemia
- » Steatorrhea

Easy acronym to remember highlights of pancreatitis:

P = PaO_2 (< 60, ARDS)

A = Age (> 55 y.o.)

N = Neutrophils (Increased WBCs)

C = Calcium (Hypocalcemia)

R = Renal function (Increased BUN)

E = Enzymes (Elevated ALT/LDH)

A = Albumin (hypoalbuminemia)

S = Sugar (Hyperglycemia)

Diagnostics

- » Labs
- » CT scan
  - • Caution with contrast; high risk renal failure

- » Ultrasound
  - • Assess for gall stones & pancreatic fluid collections
  - • If gallstone obstruction— ERCP (endoscopic retrograde cholangiopancreatography)
- » MRI
  - • Visual fluid collections or masses

Treatment

- » Supportive—multi-system organ failure
- » Rest the pancreas

- » Nutritional support, feed as soon as possible
  - • Feeding tube past the duodenum
  - • NG tube if ileus is present

» Prevent complications

» Pulmonary effusions/ARDS

» Needle aspiration of fluid—
guide antibiotic therapy

» Adequate volume resuscitation

» Pain management

Nursing interventions, monitor for:

» Respiratory compromise

» Hypovolemia

General nutrition in critically ill patients

American Society for Parenteral & Enteral Nutrition (ASPEN) Guidelines

» Minimal caloric needs:
25 kcal/kg/day

» Protein needs: 1 gram/kg/
day (bigger focus on protein)

» Assessing nutritional status

• Pre-Albumin

• Albumin

• Neither are overly helpful

» Malabsorption

» Steatorrhea—fat in stool

Bariatric Surgery

Types of Procedures:

» Adjustable Gastric Banding

» Gastric Sleeve (aka Vertical
Sleeve Gastrectomy)

» Gastric Bypass (Roux-en-Y)—
considered the "Gold Standard"
of Bariatric Surgery

» Bilio-Pancreatic Duodenal
Switch—rare

Gastric Sleeve

» Usually Laparoscopic

» 2/3 of stomach is removed

» Stomach becomes tube shaped with restriction at the proximal end

» Inner diameter—16 mm

» Monitor for bleeding & leak

Gastric Bypass (Roux-en-Y)

» Laparoscopic or open

» Create a "pouch" at the upper portion of the stomach

» Small intestine anastomosed to "pouch"

» Pouch only holds ~30 cc

» Initial rapid weight loss

» Monitor for bleeding & leak

» Many experience remission from Type 2 diabetes

Post-Op concerns

» Monitor for signs of bleeding

  • Increased HR, decreased BP

» Monitor for signs of leaking

  • SIRS, signs of sepsis

» High risk for DVT, pulmonary embolism

  • Mobilize as soon as possible!

» Monitor for hypoglycemia

» Small, frequent, usually liquid or soft meals for 1st week

» Protein based

» Long term:

  • Dumping syndrome

  • Vitamin deficiencies

  • Lactose intolerance

You can do it!

Hematology & Immunology Review

AACN Blueprint for the Hematology & Immunology portion of the CCRN® Exam

- ▶ Anemia
- ▶ Coagulopathies
- ▶ ITP, DIC, HIT
- ▶ Immune deficiencies
- ▶ Leukopenia
- ▶ Thrombocytopenia

Anemia

Who's at Risk?

» Anyone in the ICU > 7 days

» Defined Hgb < 12 g/dL for females & < 13.5 for males

  * Source: American Society of Hematology

» Reasons for anemia:

  * Frequent phlebotomy

  * Systemic inflammation

  * Loss—bleeding

  * ↓ RBC production

  * Iron &/or vitamin B_{12} deficiency

  * Chronic illness

» RBC production is regulated by erythropoietin

» Transfusion threshold.... It depends!!!

» Generally hemoglobin < 7 g/dL, Hematocrit < 21% if the patient is stable

  * Hint: Hemoglobin level multiplied by 3 gives you a hematocrit level

  * If a patient is actively bleeding, don't wait until the Hct is < 21 to transfuse!

  * In actively bleeding patients the transfusion threshold is much higher

In general...

» Anemia is tolerated as long as intravascular volume is adequate

» Hemoglobin & hematocrit tell you very little about oxygen utilization!

» All they tell you is how many cells the patient has

WBCs—Normal 5K – 10K/mm^3

Differential:

» **Neutrophils:** Normal is
55 – 70% of total WBCs

  * Primary responder to
    infection & inflammation

  * Immature neutrophils are called
    bands (3 – 6% is normal)

  * Neutropenia—decreased
    number of neutrophils;
    high risk for infection!

» **Monocytes:** Normal is
2 – 8% of total WBCs

  * Big phagocytes that mature
    into macrophages

  * Scavengers of bacteria

» **Lymphocytes:** Normal is
20 – 40% of total WBCs

  * Responsible for adaptive
    immune response

  * CD4 count is a subset, which
    is monitored in HIV

» **Eosinophils:** Normal is
1 – 4% of total WBCs

  * Increase with parasitic infections

  * Will be elevated in
    allergic response

Leukocytosis

» Elevation of WBCs (specifically
neutrophils) in response to
infection or inflammation

» Elevated WBCs are good because
they phagocytose bacteria

» Bad because neutrophils release
O_2 free radicals & excessive
cytokines from macrophages

Leukopenia

» Decrease in the number of WBCs

» See in infection with rapid
consumption of WBCs

» Increased risk of infection
& immune compromise

» Wash your hands & protect
the patient from infection!

Platelets

» Normal 150,000 – 400,000/uL

» Also called thrombocytes d/t their role in clotting

» ~65% of platelets circulate in blood, ~35% stored in spleen

Coagulopathies & Platelet Disorders

» In thrombocytopenia, either there are not enough platelets or the platelet function is impaired

» Life span of a platelet is 10 days

» Any endothelial damage causes platelets to adhere to collagen

Clot formation process:

Release of calcium →

Activation of Glycoprotein IIb/IIIa receptors on the surface of platelets →

» GP IIb/IIIa receptors bind to fibrinogen to form bridges to other platelets to form clots →

» Calcium activates the coagulation cascade

» End result → thrombus

Thrombocytopenia

» Platelet count < 150,000 /uL

» The body can form platelet plugs until the platelet count is about 100,000 /uL

» Without a structural lesion, we can tolerate platelet count ~ 5,000 /uL as long as there is no major bleeding!

» In ICUs, the incidence of thrombocytopenia is up to 35%

» Causes of thrombocytopenia:

   • Sepsis—Phagocytosis of platelets by macrophages

   • DIC

   • Inflammation

Many medications cause impaired platelet function.

Here's a short list:

» ASA

» Clopidogrel

» Prasugrel

» Pradaxa

» Glycoprotein inhibitors

» Ticlidopine

» Alteplase

» Heparin

» Dextran

» Penicillins

» Cephalosporins

» Diphenhydramine

» Calcium channel blockers

» Nitroglycerin

» Nitroprusside

» Haloperidol

» Ketorolac

Idiopathic thrombocytopenia purpura (ITP)

» Autoimmune disorder

» Destruction of platelets in spleen

» Platelet counts drop
  to < 20,000 /uL

» It is a primary disorder or a
  secondary disorder due to:

  • Medications

  • Autoimmune disorders (i.e.
    systemic lupus erythematosus)

Symptoms:

» Petechiae, purpura,
  epistaxis, splenomegaly

Treatment:

» Steroids

» Immunoglobin IV

» Monoclonal antibody therapy

» Splenectomy

Disseminated Intravascular Coagulation (DIC)

The other name for DIC is "Consumptive Coagulopathy"

» Advanced DIC has a mortality up to 80%

» Hypercoagulation secondary to widespread endothelial damage

» Microvascular thrombus formation caused by some predisposing factor like:

  • Trauma

  • Sepsis/infection

• Obstetric complications

» Release of proinflammtory cytokines → activate the clotting cascade

» Intravascular fibrin formation (micro-emboli)

» Bottom line - use up all the clotting factors, then patients bleed!

Clinical Presentation

» Tissue & organ ischemia, infarction, organ dysfunction

» Ischemic changes in hands & feet

» Bleeding or oozing from multiple sites in the body

• Petechiae

• Ecchymosis & symmetrical necrosis of limbs

• Purpura Fulminans (blood spots, bruising of skin)

• Gums, mucous membranes, nose

• Oozing from IV sites

Diagnosis

» Predisposing condition

» Lab values indicate widespread coagulation deficits

» ↓ Platelets; often less than 50,000

» ↑ D-dimer; 1 – 5 mcg/mL, advanced > 5 mcg/mL (normal is < 0.4 mcg/mL)

» ↓ Fibrinogen; < 100 mg/dL (normal is 200 – 400 mg/dL)

» ↓ Prothrombin Index; 40 – 70, advanced < 40

» ↑ aPTT/PT/INR

Treatment:

» Treat the cause (i.e. sepsis, trauma, obstetric emergency)

» Supportive

» Volume replacement

» Treat bleeding:
  * Platelet transfusions
  * Cryoprecipitate

Heparin Induced Thrombocytopenia (HIT)

» Platelet count drops by ≥ 50% within 5 – 10 days of exposure to heparin

» May develop more quickly if previous exposure to heparin

» Erythematous lesions around SQ Heparin injection sites

» 25% of patients develop systemic reaction
  * Fever
  * Chills
  * Tachypnea
  * Tachycardia
  * Generally not associated with bleeding

» **Major Complication: Thrombosis
  * 75% of cases develop systemic thrombosis
  * 50% DVT of lower extremity
  * 10% DVT of upper extremity
  * 25% Pulmonary embolus
  * Arterial thrombosis
  * AMI & Stroke

» Risk is greater with unfractionated heparin (UFH)

» Even low doses & heparin flushes

» Don't forget: heparin coated catheters

Diagnosis of HIT:

» Clinical exposure to heparin

» Thrombocytopenia

» Symptomatic thrombosis

» IGG antibodies to heparin

  * Platelet factor 4 complex
  * Antibody assay

» Clinical picture + assay for diagnosis

Treatment of HIT:

» Discontinue all forms of heparin!!!

Anticoagulation using Direct Thrombin Inhibitors (DTIs):

» Angiomax (Bivalirudin)

  * Initial: 0.15 - 0.2 mg/kg/hr IV

  * Adjust to aPTT 1.5 - 2.5 times baseline value

  * Renal adjustments are necessary

» Argatroban

  * Cleared by the liver

  * 2 mcg/kg/min – Max 10 mcg/kg/min

  * PTT 1.5 – 3 x baseline value, not to exceed 100 seconds

» Long term anticoagulation with Coumadin

  * HOWEVER, do not use during the active phase of HIT

  * Increased risk of limb gangrene

» Heparin antibodies last > 100 days after exposure

» Do not reintroduce heparin as long as antibodies persist!

Commonly used anticoagulants

Coumadin (warfarin)

» Acts on extrinsic & common coagulation pathways

» Monitor PT/INR

» Therapeutic goal INR 2 – 3x baseline

  * DVT prophylaxis

  * PE prophylaxis/treatment

  * Atrial fibrillation

» Therapeutic goal INR 2.5 – 3.5x baseline

  * Mechanical prosthetic valves

» To reverse warfarin:

  * Vitamin K (phytonadione) 2.5 – 5 mg PO

  * 1 – 2.5 mg IV SLOWLY over an hour

  * Will see INR drop within 8 – 12 hours

» Serious or life threatening bleeding

  * Vitamin K 10 mg IV SLOWLY— never give IV push!

  * Fresh Frozen Plasma (FFP)

» Prothrombin Complex
Concentrate (PCC)

» NovoSeven—recombinant
factor seven

Heparin (unfractionated)

» Acts on intrinsic & common
coagulation pathways

» Monitor aPTT

- Normal 25 – 38 seconds

- Can also monitor Factor Xa levels

» For procedural sheath removal,
can also monitor ACT

- Therapeutic ACT 300
– 350 seconds

- Discontinue sheath when
ACT < 150 seconds

» Heparin reversal:
Protamine sulfate

Protamine sulfate for anticoagulation reversal

» Heparin reversal: 1 – 1.5
mg of Protamine per
100 units of Heparin

- Do not exceed 50 mg
Protamine IV

» Dalteparin reversal: 1 mg of
Protamine per 100 units of
Dalteparin administered

» Enoxaparin reversal: 1 mg
of Protamine per 1 mg of
enoxaparin if enoxaparin
given within 8 hours

» Adverse effects of Protamine:

- Hypotension

- Nausea/vomiting

- Anaphylaxis

Low Molecular Weight Heparin vs. Unfractionated Heparin

Benefits of LMWH:

» Less incidence of HIT

» No need to monitor aPTT

» Longer half-life

- 4 – 6 hours vs. 1 – 2 hours

» More predictable d/t
bioavailability

- 90% bioavailable vs.
30% with UFH

Novel Oral Anticoagulation (NOACs)—mostly FYI

» Pradaxa (dabigatran)

- Used for non-valvular atrial fibrillation, VTE prophylaxis
- Half-life 12 – 14 hours
- Praxbind is the reversal agent for bleeding
- Currently, no other NOAC has a reversal agent

» Xarelto (rivaroxaban)— Direct Factor Xa Inhibitor

- Used for non-valvular afib, VTE prevention

» Savaysa, Lixiana (edoxaban)— Direct Factor Xa Inhibitor

- Used for VTE prophylaxis after ortho surgery, stroke prevention

» Eliquis (apixiban)—Direct Factor Xa Inhibitor

- Used to prevent venous thromboembolic events

» Reversal:

- If ingested in < 2 hours, activated charcoal
- Otherwise, control bleeding

Blood Products

» Whole blood is rarely used; it's inefficient

» It is spun down via centrifuge to:

- Erythrocytes & plasma

» PRBCs

- 200 mLs of cells
- 50 – 100 mLs of CPD & plasma

» Order leukocyte— reduced PRBCs if:

- History of febrile hemolytic transfusion reactions
- 30% of leukocytes still remain even if leuko-reduced
- Many blood banks are leuko-reducing PRBCs

» Washed RBCs

- Reduce leukocytes & plasma
- Reduces reactions from plasma proteins

» The universal donor is O Negative

» Universal recipient is AB

» Only use normal saline with transfusions...why not Lactated Ringers?

- LR contains calcium that can promote clotting!!!

Platelet Transfusions

» When whole blood is donated, platelets get separated with leukocytes

* Increased incidence of fever with platelet transfusion d/t leukocytes

» Banked platelets are usually pooled

» Store banked platelets up to 7 days

» Viability decreases after 3 days

» When a 6 pack platelets is transfused:

* 30,000/uL rise

* See increase 1 hour after transfusion, lasts up to 8 days

» If not seeing an increase in the platelet count with a transfusion consider:

* Leukocyte reduced transfusion

* ABO compatibility

PRBCs

» Stored at 4°C – 21 day shelf life

» CPD preservative

* **C**itrate

  ▷ Binds to calcium— anticoagulant

  ▷ Monitor calcium levels when transfusing PRBCs. They can get hypocalcemic!

  ▷ Patient will need 500—1 Gram of Ca^{++} for every 3 – 4 units of PRBCs

* **P**hosphate

  ▷ Slows breakdown of 2,3-DPG; banked blood low in 2,3-DPG

  ▷ 2,3 DPG encourages unloading between O_2 & hemoglobin

* **D**extrose

  ▷ Fuel source for blood cells

Hemolytic Reactions

» Usually human error

» Can also be ABO compatibility

» It only take about 5 mLs to see a reaction

» Signs:

- Fever

- Tachycardia or bradycardia

- Dyspnea

- Chest pain

- Low back pain

- Hypotension

- Blood in urine

Treatment:

» Stop the transfusion immediately!!!

- Morbidity & mortality is r/t the amount of blood received

» Monitor vital signs

» Infuse fluids—support BP

» Send unit to the Blood Bank

» Coomb's Test—Positive reaction if there is a hemolytic reaction

You can do it!

Multi-System Review

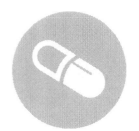

AACN Blueprint for the Multi-System portion of the CCRN® Exam

- Bariatric complications
- Comorbidity in patients with transplant history
- End of life
- Healthcare associated infections
- CLABSI
- CAUTI
- VAP (VAE)—covered in Pulmonary section
- Hypotension
- Infections
- Multi-organ dysfunction (MODS)
- Multisystem Trauma
- Pain
- Palliative care
- Rhabdomyolysis
- Sepsis continuum
- Shock states
- Sleep disruption
- Thermoregulation
- Toxin/drug exposure
- Toxic Ingestions (Drug/ETOH overdose)

Behavioral/Psychosocial

- Agitation
- Antisocial behaviors, aggression, violence
- Delirium
- Dementia
- Medical non-adherence
- Mood disorders, depression, anxiety
- Post-traumatic stress disorder (PTSD)
- Risk-taking behavior
- Substance dependence (i.e. ETOH withdrawal, drug seeking behavior, chronic alcohol or drug dependence)
- Suicidal ideation and/or behaviors

Integumentary

- IV infiltration
- Pressure ulcers
- Wounds (infectious, surgical, trauma)

Sepsis

Early Recognition is Key!!!

» **S**ystemic **I**nflammatory **R**esponse **S**yndrome **(SIRS):**

» ≥ 2 of the following:

* Temperature > 38.3°C (100.9°F) or < 36°C (96.8°F)

* Heart rate > 90 bpm
* RR > 20 bpm or $PaCO_2$ < 32
* WBC > 12,000 or < 4,000 or > 10% band forms

If a patient meets SIRS criteria, do you suspect an infection?

Note: SIRS is also seen in sepsis, burns, trauma, surgery, autoimmune disorders, pancreatitis…so, it is sensitive, but not specific to sepsis!

Definitions of Sepsis

» Sepsis: SIRS + infection

» Severe Sepsis: Sepsis + Organ dysfunction

» Septic Shock: Severe Sepsis + either: SBP < 90, MAP < 65, or lactate > 4 after fluids

* Severe sepsis + refractory hypotension = Septic shock
* Abnormal function of > 1 organ = **M**ulti-**O**rgan **D**ysfunction (MODS)

Common organ involvement:

» Lungs

* Monitor for increasing O_2 needs or difficulty breathing

» Kidneys

* Monitor urine output

» Cardiovascular system

* Monitor signs of decreased C.O., hypotension

» Central nervous system

* Watch for confusion or LOC changes

Tissue hypoxia caused by cardiovascular abnormalities

» Vasodilation

» Capillary leak

» Formation of micro-emboli

» Release of myocardial depressant factor

Leads to:

» Decreased intravascular volume

» Tissue edema

» Poor O_2 diffusion

» Poor O_2 unloading to the tissues

Signs of acute organ dysfunction:

» Altered consciousness, confusion, psychosis

» Tachypnea, PaO_2 < 70 mm Hg, SaO_2 < 90%, PaO_2/FiO_2 ≤ 300

» Jaundice, ↑ LFTs, ↑ bilirubin, ↓ albumin, ↑PT/INR

» Tachycardia, hypotension, altered CVP, altered PAOP

» Oliguria, anuria, ↑ creatinine

» ↓ Platelets, ↓protein C, ↑ D-dimer

2015—3 & 6 Hour Sepsis Bundle

Early detection—1st 3 hours

» Measure lactate level

» Obtain blood cultures prior to administration of antibiotics

» Administer broad spectrum antibiotics

» Administer 30 ml/kg crystalloid for hypotension or lactate ≥ 4 mmol/L

Critical Care—1st 6 hours

» Apply vasopressors for hypotension (that does not respond to fluid resuscitation) to maintain MAP ≥ 65 mm Hg

- Norepinephrine infusion

- Vasopressin infusion (2nd line agent)

» For persistent hypotension after initial fluid administration, or if initial lactate was ≥ 4 mmol/L, reassess volume status & tissue perfusion

» Re-measure lactate if initial was elevated

SEP-1 Measure (from the CORE measure)

Document reassessment of volume status and tissue perfusion with either:

» Repeat focused exam (after initial fluid resuscitation) by licensed independent practitioner including vital signs, cardiopulmonary, capillary refill, pulse and skin findings

Or two of the following:

» Measure CVP

» Measure $ScvO_2$

» Bedside cardiovascular ultrasound

» Dynamic assessment of fluid responsiveness with passive leg raise or fluid challenge

Lactate

» In sepsis, lactate should be viewed as a marker of tissue perfusion

» Lactate has some prognostic utility

» Sustained elevated lactate > 6 hours portends increased mortality

» Mortality increases as lactate levels increase

* 0 – 2.5 mmol/L   4.9% mortality

* 2.5 – 4.0 mmol/L   9.0%

* > 4.0 mmol/L   28.4%

Lactate Clearance

» Re-measure lactate after fluids

» It should decrease; ideally by at least 10% with each fluid bolus

» The goals is always to normalize the lactate

SvO$_2$ / ScvO$_2$:

» SvO$_2$ Goal > 60 – 75%

* Measured with a pulmonary artery catheter

* "True" mixed venous

» ScvO$_2$ Goal > 70%

* Surrogate of mixed venous (SvO$_2$)

* Measured continuously with a specific central line

* Can also measure intermittently via central line or PICC line

* 5 – 8% higher than SvO$_2$

Sepsis key points...

» <u>Early</u> recognition

» In the 1st 3 hours:

* Labs – Lactate, CBC with differential, cultures

* Fluids (30 ml/kg to start)

* Repeat lactate after fluid boluses

* Antibiotics: Broad spectrum, then narrow

* Source control

* Prevent critical care!!!

Anaphylaxis

» Inflammatory response &
hypersensitivity reaction

Common allergens:

» Contrast dye

» Food

» Antimicrobials

» Insect bites

» Symptoms minutes to hours

Less serious reactions:

» Flushing, erythema, rash,
urticaria, diarrhea

More serious:

» Angioedema, laryngeal
edema, tongue swelling,
bronchospasm, hypotension

Anaphylaxis treatment:

1st Line Treatment:

» Monitor airway!!!

» Epinephrine 1:1,000 strength

» 0.3 mg IM

» Blocks the release of
inflammatory mediators

» Can also nebulize the
epinephrine to treat
laryngeal edema

» If taking a beta blocker, can
give Glucagon 5 – 15 mcg/
min IV continuous infusion

2nd Line Treatment: (Histamine blockers)

» Diphenhydramine 25
  – 50 mg IV/IM/PO

  * H_1 blocker

» Ranitidine 50 mg IV or 150 mg PO

  * H_2 blocker

» Synergistic effect

» Steroids—prevent 2nd
  phase symptoms

  * Prednisone 50 mg PO <u>or</u>

  * Methylprednisolone 125 mg IV

» If progression to
  anaphylactic shock:

  * Massive vasodilation
    with fluid shifts

  * Decrease afterload & preload

  * Volume resuscitation

  * Consider colloids

» For refractory hypotension:

  * Vasoconstrictors to "tighten
    up" vasculature

    ▷ Epinephrine infusion 2 – 8
      mcg/min

    ▷ Dopamine infusion 5 – 20
      mcg/kg/min

    ▷ Norepinephrine infusion 2 –
      8 mcg/min

Overdoses

Acetaminophen Overdose:

» Included in over 600
  drug preparations

» Leading cause of toxic
  ingestions & acute liver failure

» Over 1/3 are unintentional

» 80 – 90% metabolized
  through the liver

» Toxic metabolite accumulates
  & causes widespread
  hepatocellular damage

Risk Assessment:

» Determine ingested dose—amount & time

» 7.5 to 15 grams can cause toxicity

» Concomitant use of ETOH increases risk

» Assess plasma acetaminophen levels

* Measure 4 – 24° after ingestion to predict risk

» If the level falls in the high risk category of nomogram, risk of hepatotoxicity is ≥ 60%

4 Stages of Toxicity:

1st 24 hours after ingestion:

» No or vague symptoms

» No lab value / evidence of injury

24 – 72 hours:

» No or vague symptoms

» ↑ AST—most sensitive

» Precedes hepatic dysfunction

72 – 96 hours:

» Progressive hepatic injury

» Peak AST levels

» Encephalopathy

» Coagulopathy

» Renal insufficiency

3 – 5 days:

» Start recovery or death

Treatment:

- » Antidote: N-Acetylcysteine (Mucomyst)
  - Goal: Limit accumulation of the metabolite to prevent hepatocellular damage
    - Ideal to start within 24 hours of ingestion
    - IV preferred d/t smell
- » Activated charcoal is also an option if used within 4 hours of ingestion

N-Acetylcysteine dosing:

- » IV dosing: 150 mg/kg over 60 min
  - 50 mg/kg over 4 hrs, then 100 mg/kg over 16 hrs
  - Total: 300 mg/kg over 21 hrs
- » PO dosing: 140 mg/kg PO load, then 70 mg/kg Q 4 hours
  - Total: 1330 mg/kg over 72 hrs

Benzodiazepine Overdose:

- » 2nd most common overdose in the US
- » Usually involve a 2nd respiratory depressant

Higher risk:

- » Advanced age
- » Accumulative dosing
- » Assess for concomitant use with opioids

Treatment:

**Antagonist: Flumazenil (Romazicon)

- » IV - 0.2 mg repeated Q 1 – 6 min up to 1 mg
  - Onset: 1 – 2 min
  - Peak: 6 – 10 min
  - Duration: 60 min
- » Duration of benzos often last longer than the antidote
- » Monitor for re-sedation

» Can do continuous Romazicon infusion 0.3 – 0.4 mg/hr

» Monitor for benzo withdrawal; seizure precautions

Aspirin (Salicylate) Overdose:

Diagnosis:

» Clinical presentation

» Anion gap (+ gap)

» ABGs

» Respiratory alkalosis d/t brain stimulation of respiratory center

» Monitor serum salicylate levels

» Acute ingestion of > 150 mg/kg can cause severe toxicity

» Salicylate tablets may form bezoars, prolonging absorption and toxicity

  • Need to know if enteric coated

Signs:

» Vomiting

» Tinnitus

» Confusion

» Hyperthermia

» Irregular breathing patterns

» Metabolic acidosis

» Multiple organ failure

Treatment:

» Activated charcoal

» Bicarb infusion

» Alkaline diuresis

» IV fluids

» Hemodialysis

» Supportive

Opioid Overdose:

» Morphine most common in hospitalized patients

» Heroin for street drugs

Treatment:

Antagonist: Naloxone

» Binds to opioid receptors

» Dose: 0.4 mg IV or IM

* Onset IV: 2 - 3 min, IM 5 - 15 min

* Repeat in 2 min up to 1 mg

* Opioid dependency dose 0.1 – 0.2 mg

» Monitor for recurrent respiratory depression

* 2 mg IV; repeat Q 2 min up to 10 mg

* Effects last 60 min

* Can also consider an infusion

Adverse effects of Naloxone:

» Anxiety

» Abdominal cramping

» N/V

» Piloerection

Beta Blocker Overdose:

» Over 15 FDA approved in the US

Side effects:

» Bradycardia

» Hypotension (d/t vasodilation & renin blockade)

» Decreased C.O.

» B_1 receptor blockade

» Heart block from prolonged A-V conduction

Neurotoxicity:

» Lethargy, ↓ LOC, seizures

» Seizures more common with Propranolol

Antidote: Glucagon

» 3 mg IV initial dose (0.05 mcg/kg)

» 5 mg IV repeated dose (0.07 mcg/kg)

» Continuous infusion 5 mg/hr if needed

» Reverses the B_1 blockade

» Mimics + inotropic effects of beta receptor activation

» Atropine may be needed for the bradycardia

  * Give the Glucagon first
  * Prepare to emergently pace

Side effects of Glucagon:

» N/V

» Mild hyperglycemia

» Hypokalemia

» Hypertension

Calcium Channel Blocker Overdose:

» Over 10 FDA approved

» Verapamil, nifedipine & diltiazem most common

» Ca^{++} influx into myocardial cell is essential & determines strength of contraction

Effects:

» Negative inotropic effects (reduces C.O.)

» Negative chronotropic effects (bradycardia)

» Prolonged AV conduction

» Vasodilation

» Bronchial dilation

Neuro effects:

- » Lethargy

- » ↓ LOC

- » Generalized seizures

- » Hyperglycemia (inhibits insulin release)

Treatment:

- » Calcium!!!

- » Calcium chloride 10% IV

  - ∗ 1 amp = 1.36 mEq/ml

  - ∗ Prevent blockade – 3 ml

  - ∗ Reverse blockade – 10 ml/13.6 mEq

- » Calcium gluconate 10% IV

  - ∗ 1 amp = 0.46 mEq/ml

  - ∗ Prevent blockade – 10 ml

  - ∗ Reverse blockade – 30 ml/13.8 mEq

- » Can use continuous IV since effects are so short lived (10 – 15 min)

  - ∗ 0.3 – 0.7 mEq/kg/hr

- » Atropine 0.5 – 1.0 mg IV

  - ∗ Reverse bradycardia

  - ∗ Give Ca^{++} first!!!

  - ∗ Atropine is enhanced by calcium administration

- » If continued hypotension, use catecholamine infusion:

  - ∗ Epinephrine, norepinephrine or dopamine

ETOH Withdrawal

- » Potentially life threatening

- » <u>Sudden</u> cessation of alcohol intake or reduced consumption

- » Symptoms can start as early as 2 hours & continue for weeks

Symptoms of withdrawal:

- » Tachycardia

- » Tachypnea

- » Tremors

- » Anxiety

- » Irritation

- » Sweating

- » Seizures

- » DTs—delirium tremens

Clinical Institute Withdrawal Assessment Scale (CIWA) assesses:

» Nausea & vomiting

» Paroxysmal sweating

» Agitation

» Visual disturbances

» Tremor

» Tactile disturbances

» Headache

» Auditory disturbances

» Orientation/clouding sensorium

Scoring:

» < 8: No medications needed

» 9 – 14: Optional medications

» 15 – 19: Give medication

» 20: High risk for complications

Treatment of DTs

Pharmacologic:

» Benzodiazepines
  • Lorazepam

» Librium

» Dexmetomidine (Precedex)
  • Monitor for bradycardia

» Low dose anti-psychotics
  • Haldol
  • Quetiapine (Seroquel)

  • Monitor for prolonged QTc interval

» IV fluids

» Electrolyte imbalance (Mg^{++})

» Thiamine

» Anti-seizure medications
  • Prophylactic if previous seizures from withdrawal

Nursing:

» Safety

» Quiet environment

» Airway

» Seizure precautions

» Cardiac monitoring

» Monitor QTc if giving anti-psychotics

» In general, elderly at higher risk

Delirium

» Acute brain dysfunction

» Key characteristics:

* Inattention

* Confusion

* Disorganized thinking

* Can wax & wane

* Hyperactive & hypoactive

Who is at risk?

» Hospitalized patients

» Elderly

» Stroke, CNS issues

» Sepsis

» Sleep deprived

» Electrolyte imbalances

» Dehydration

» Memory impaired

» Severe burns or trauma

Monitoring for delirium

» Confusion Assessment Method (CAM)—ICU Assessment

» Most validated tool & widely used

» Assess for fluctuation in neuro status from baseline

» Assess RASS (or sedation level)

PAD Guidelines

» Guidelines to give direction
on how to prevent and
manage delirium

Pain

» Treat pain first!!!

» Use a behavioral pain
assessment scale

» Ask the right questions

» Do not use sedatives to treat pain

» Pre-emptive pain plan for:
  * Treatments
  * Mobility
  * Dressing changes

Agitation

» Minimize sedation

» Avoid benzodiazepines
  * Unless ETOH withdrawal

» Consider non-benzodiazepines
for sedation if needed
  * Propofol
  * Dexmetomidine (Precedex)

» Don't overuse sedation;
"light" sedation
  * RASS—1 to 0 should be the goal

» Avoid "deep" sedation unless
absolutely clinically warranted

» Daily interruption in
sedation (wake patient up)

» Determine sedation goal

» Remove any unnecessary
lines or tubes

» Consider non-pharmacologic
interventions

Delirium

» Prevent it!!!

» Monitor for it!!!

» Identify who is at risk

» If the patient develops delirium:

 * Identify reversible causes:

   T = Toxins

   H = Hypoxemia

   I = Infection

   N = Non-pharmacologic interventions

   K = K$^+$ (electrolyte imbalances— Na$^+$ is a big one!)

 * Avoid benzodiazepines

 * Dexmetomidine (Precedex) associated with lower delirium risk vs. benzo

» Review the medication list—eliminate any meds not necessary

» Pharmacist consult

General prevention considerations:

» Glasses & hearing aids on/in the patient!

» Day/night orientation

» Method of communicating if barrier

» Frequent reorientation

» Mobility!

» Board in room with place & date

» Clock in view

» Noise control

» Promote sleep

» Cluster care activities

You can do it!

Neurology Review

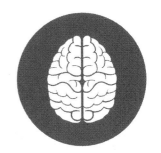

AACN Blueprint for the Neurology portion of the CCRN® Exam

- Brain Death
- Encephalopathy (anoxic, hypoxic-ischemic)
- Hemorrhage (ICH, IVH, Subarachnoid)
- Ischemic stroke
- Neuro Infectious Disease
- Neurosurgery
- Seizure Disorders
- Space Occupying Lesions (tumors)
- Traumatic brain injury (epidural, subdural, concussion, non-accidental)

Brain anatomy & function

» Frontal lobe:

* Personality, motor function, motor speech, morals, emotions, judgment

» Parietal lobe:

* Sensation, pain interpretation, temperature, pressure

» Temporal lobe:

* Auditory & speech

» Occipital lobe:

* Visual

» Cerebellum:

* Coordination of muscle movement & tone, coordination, equilibrium

» Brain Stem:

* Basic functions—breathing

4 Ventricles:

» Two lateral ventricles

» Foramen of Monro:

* Conduit of CSF flow from the lateral ventricles to the third ventricle

» Third & Fourth Ventricles

Cerebral Spinal Fluid (CSF)

» Clear, colorless

» Large amount of NaCl, some protein & glucose

» Cushions and protects the brain & spinal cord

» 500 ml produced per day

Intracranial Pressure (ICP)

» Brain compartment is comprised of:

* 80% Tissue

* 10% CSF

* 10% Blood

Monro-Kellie Doctrine:

» Balance of tissue, CSF & blood to create an equilibrium

» Increase in one area must result in a decrease in another

» If not, the ICP will increase

* Compression of venous blood

* Displacement of CSF

* Blood flow is maintained by cerebral auto-regulation

Causes of Intracranial Hypertension:

» Trauma—TBI

» Intracranial Hemorrhage

» Hydrocephalus

» Cerebral edema

» Stroke

» Brain tumors

» Hypoxic-ischemic brain injury (cardiac arrest)

» Brain infections/abscess

» Fever

» Seizures

External Causes of Intracranial Hypertension:

» Suctioning

» Position changes

» Nursing care

» Positive End-Expiratory Pressure (PEEP)

» Increased stimuli

Neuro Assessment

» Level of consciousness

» Mentation: Are there changes? Even slight?

» Pupillary response: Equal & reactive?

» Motor skills: Equal on both sides?

* Against resistance?

» Sensory deficits?

* Test with light touch/pinprick

» Vision or speech deficits?

» Cranial Nerve Assessment

» Glasgow Coma Scale measures:

- Best eye response
- Best verbal response
- Best motor response

Signs of Increased ICP

» **Change in LOC

» Headache

» Nausea/vomiting

- Can progress to projectile

» Lethargy

» Irritability

» Slow decision making

Late changes:

» Pupillary changes

» Dilation in one eye

» Seizures

» Posturing

» Can progress to coma

Monitoring Intracranial Pressure (ICP)

Who should be monitored?

» Early recognition of changes in ICP

» Head injuries—GCS < 8

» Cerebral edema

» Large ischemic stroke with potential ICP issues

» Hydrocephalus

ICP Parameters

» Normal ICP 0 – 15 mm Hg

» Treatment indicated if sustained > 20 – 25 mm Hg

» Calculate Cerebral Perfusion Pressure (CPP)

  • MAP – ICP = CPP

  • Goal > 60 (Usually 70 – 90)

Methods of monitoring ICP

» Intra-ventricular catheter

  • Used to drain excessive CSF & intermittently monitor ICP

» Intraparenchymal

  • Monitor pressure only

  • Commonly referred to as a "bolt"

What's in an ICP waveform?

» P1—Percussion wave

» P2—Tidal Wave

» P3—Dicrotic notch (closure of aortic valve)

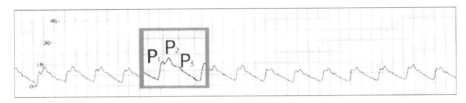

» What is the significance of an elevated P2 wave?

  • Decreased compliance!

Managing increased ICP

First Tier Interventions:

» Patient positioning

  • Manage venous drainage

» Prevent compression of jugular veins

» HOB 30 – 45 degrees

» Good head alignment— keep midline

» Straight legs

» Decrease stimuli

» Analgesics—assess for pain

» Normothermia

- Fever associated with worse outcomes

Second Tier Interventions:

» Mannitol 20% - Osmotic diuretic

- 0.25 to 1 gram/kg IV bolus
- ICP decrease within 5 – 10 min
- Maximum effect in 1 hour
- Use filter!
- May repeat q 1 – 4 hours

» Hypertonic Saline (2%, 3%, 5%)

- Continuous infusion
- Monitor osmolality & Na^+ levels

» Loop Diuretics

- Decrease intracranial blood volume

» Considerations for all:

- Monitor serum osmo & fluid status
- OSMO no higher than 320 mOsm/L
  - ▷ Or patient specific goal
- Monitor for rebound increase in ICPs
- Potassium levels (can get hypokalemic)
- Keep CPP > 60 mm Hg

» Sedation

- Propofol (if intubated)
- Use only short acting sedatives

» Mild hyperventilation in mechanically ventilated patients

- Low normal $PaCO_2$ 35 – 40 mm Hg
- Decreased $PaCO_2$ causes vasoconstriction

» Barbiturate coma

- Pentobarbital
  - ▷ Closely monitor for hypotension
  - ▷ Use continuous EEG
- Thiopental

» Neuromuscular blockade (NMB)

- Must ALWAYS be intubated & used with continuous IV sedation
- Assess peripheral nerve stimulation to assess dosing
- Goal 1—2 twitches out of 4
- Protect the corneas with lubricant

» With NMB, what is the significance of having:

» 0 / 4 twitches?

* Need to decrease dose of NMB

» 4 / 4 twitches?

* Need to increase dose of NMB

» Decompressive Craniectomy

* Used for refractory intracranial hypertension when other approaches have failed

Traumatic Brain Injuries (TBI)

Types

» Blunt

» Penetrating

» Blast

Focal

» Coup-countrecoup

» Contusions

» Lacerations

» Arterial or venous tears

Causes

» Motor Vehicle Crash

» Assault

» Falls

Diffuse Brain Injuries "Shearing injury"

» Twist & turn of axons/ shearing injury

» Mild—concussion

* Usually < 15 min alteration in LOC

* Stretch injury of the axons

* Attention span & memory affected (cortical function)

* Confusion & disorientation after injury

- Symptoms usually cease after 15 – 30 min
- Nausea, vomiting, dizziness, headache
- Can last for a few days

» Severe—Diffuse Axonal Injury

- Acceleration/deceleration injury
- Damage to axons

- Disconnects the cerebral hemisphere from the reticular activating system (RAS)
- Coma, often involves the brainstem
- Increased ICP
- Cerebral edema
- Fever
- Poor prognosis

Skull Fractures

Signs of a skull fracture:

» Headache

» Nausea/vomiting

» Blurred vision

» Restlessness, irritability

» Disequilibrium

» Nuchal rigidity—stiff neck

» Pupils sluggish or not reacting to light

» Confusion

» Drowsiness

Key assessment: Is the dura torn?

» CT Scan (most common) or MRI

- Yes → surgery to remove bone fragments

» Monitor for CSF leak

» High risk of infection

Types of skull fractures:

Linear skull fracture

» No treatment required

» Dura usually intact

Depressed skull fracture

» If less than thickness of the skull, no intervention

» If > thickness of skull (~6 mm), will need decompression (OR)

Basilar skull fracture

» Fracture in the floor of the skull

» Risk of injury to cranial nerves

» Avoid NASOGASTRIC or ORAL TUBES!!

  * Avoid oral suctioning

» Battle sign

  * Ecchymosis on mastoid bone

» Raccoon eyes

  * Ecchymosis around eyes

» Rhinorrhea

  * Torn blood vessels in the nose

  * CSF can leak; indicates rupture of the meninges

  * C/O salty taste (from the Na^+ in CSF)

» Otorrhea

  * Test for glucose, + glucose = CSF

  * "Halo" sign—place fluid on gauze, if iridescent halo, likely CSF

» Pneumocephalus—air in head

  * Also look for other injuries (Subdural hematoma, contusions)

  * Treatment HOB flat (if able)

  * High concentration oxygen; dissolves the air

Acute Epidural Hematoma

» Neuro emergency!!!!— arterial bleed

» Usually temporal or parietal region

» Laceration of meningeal artery &/or vein

Presentation:

- » Loss of consciousness → lucid → coma

- » Nausea, vomiting, agitation, confusion

- » Uncal (lateral) herniation

- » Pupils uneven

Subdural Hematoma (SDH)

- » Bleeding between the dura mater & the arachnoid space

- » Elderly are at risk especially if on anticoagulation

- » All types of SDH can develop spontaneously r/t anticoagulation therapy

Acute SDH

- » Symptoms hours to days

- » Decreased LOC

- » Signs of increased ICP

- » Ipsilateral occulomotor paralysis

- » Contralateral hemiparesis

Sub-acute SDH

- » Hematoma can form 2 days - 2 weeks after initial injury

Chronic SDH

- » Re-bleed weeks following injury

- » Elderly

- » Headaches

- » Confusion

Epidural & subdural hematoma diagnosis:

» CT Scan—Gold standard

» MRI—If stable

» Angiography—if arterial dissection suspected

Complications associated with TBI

» Hyponatremia

» Cerebral salt wasting

» SIADH

» Hypernatremia

» Diabetes insipidus

» Pulmonary complications/ aspiration

» Seizures

» Immobility

» DVT

Know how to monitor for each of these!

Herniation:

Signs of Supratentorial (Uncal) herniation

» Uncus pressure on the tentorial notch

» Compression of the midbrain

» Change in LOC

» Unilateral pupil dilation

» Lateral displacement

Infratentorial herniation

» Downward pressure toward brainstem & medulla

» Cushing's response:
  * Bradycardia
  * Systolic hypertension with Wide pulse pressure

* Irregular respirations

» Small pupils

» Ataxic respirations

» Coma

Posturing:

Decorticate (Flexion)

» Flexion of the arms, wrist & fingers

» Internal rotation of the lower extremities

Decerebrate (Extension)

» Arch the back

» Primitive response

» Arms extended and pronated

Brain Death Exam

» Must be normothermic

» Narcotics/sedatives cleared from system

» Absence of EEG activity

» Absence of Somatosensory Evoked Potential (SSEP)

  * Electrical signals going from the body to the brain & spinal cord

  * Identified if nerves connected to spinal cord are able to send & receive sensory information like pain, temperature and touch

» ICP > MAP

» Assess cerebral blood flow

» Evaluation of cerebral perfusion using:

  * MRI, CT angio, or Transcranial Doppler

  * Absence of cerebral blood flow

In brain death, everything is absent/negative, except the apnea test.

» Apnea test is + because the patient is apneic!

» Oculocephalic reflex (aka "doll's eyes")

  * Cranial nerves III, VI, VIII

  * Absent in brain death

  * Normal response—eyes move with head turn

» Oculovestibular Reflex
(aka "cold calorics")

- Cranial Nerves III, VI, VIII

- Absent in brain death

- Normal response—look
toward the stimulus

» Absent cough

» Absent gag

» Absent pupillary response

» Absent corneal reflex

Stroke

2 Types:

» Ischemic

- Embolic

- Thrombotic

- 85% of all strokes

- May present with transient
ischemic attack (TIA)

  ▷ Warning sign of stroke

  ▷ Blood supply to brain tissue
  briefly halting

» Hemorrhagic

AHA Stroke Guidelines

» 1 hour goals:
  - Complete National Institute
  of Health Stroke Scale
  (NIHSS) Assessment

- Treat with fibrinolytic
therapy (if appropriate)

  ▷ Embolic only

NIH Stroke Scale assesses:

» LOC

» Eye deviation (CN III, VI, VIII)

» Visual field loss (hemianopia)

» Facial palsy

» Motor arms (drift)

» Motor legs

» Limb ataxia

» Sensory

» Language

» Dysarthria

» Extinction & inattention

Diagnostics:

» CT scan <u>without</u> contrast

- R/O hemorrhage
- Should be interpreted within 45 min
- Might see hypodensity in ischemic area

» CT perfusion or MRI perfusion

- Measures infarct core or penumbra

» Non-invasive intra-cranial vascular study if plan to do intra-arterial fibrinolysis or mechanical thrombectomy

Treatment: rtPA

rtPA Considerations:

» Administer within 3 hours or,

» Extended 4.5 hour window, but excludes:

- Age > 80
- Taking oral anticoagulation
- Hx of stroke or DM
- Baseline NIHSS score > 25
- Imaging reveals ischemic injury > 1/3 of the MCA territory

» Baseline labs/tests:

- CBC, coags, chemistry with glucose, troponin, 12 lead ECG

» **Control BP prior to administration!!**

- Goal SBP < 185, DBP < 110

» Dosing rtPA: 0.9 mg/kg IV, maximum of 90 mg

- "Door to needle" time within 60 min of hospital arrival or stroke identification

» Other medication tips:

- Aspirin 325 mg should be given within 24 - 48 hours of stroke onset
- Do not provide other anticoagulation therapy within 24 hours of rtPA
- Restart statins if they were previously taking them

Endovascular therapies for ischemic stroke:

» Newer evidence to administer rtPA with endovascular procedures

» Should receive rtPA regardless

» May be reasonable in patients with a contraindication to IV fibrinolysis

» Intra-arterial rtPA may also be considered

Stroke care components:

» Cardiac monitoring

  * Atrial fibrillation & cardiac arrhythmias

» Echocardigram

  * Assess for Atrial Septal Defect (ASD) or Patent Foramen Ovale (PFO)

» Restart anti-hypertensives after 24 hours

» Airway support

  * Ventilatory assistance if needed

  * Apply O_2 if sats are < 94%

  * Aspiration risk

» Avoid fever!!! (temp > 37.5°C)

  * Antipyretic therapy

» Treat hypovolemia

» Treat hypoglycemia (< 60 mg/dL)

  * Goal: normoglycemia

  * BS 140 – 180

  * Worse outcomes if hyper or hypoglycemic

» DVT prophylaxis

  * SCDs or prophylactic anticoagulation

  * Early mobilization

» NPO until swallow evaluation

  * Nurse-driven swallow screen

  * If unable to take solids, consider placing a feeding tube

  * If > 2 weeks, consider PEG

» Avoid in-dwelling urinary catheters

  * High risk of UTIs specifically in the neuro population

Nursing considerations for stroke care:

» Frequent neuro checks

- Monitor for signs of increased ICP

- Placement of a Ventriculostomy drain if develop hydrocephalus

- Prophylactic anti-convulsants are not recommended

» Corticosteroids are not routinely recommended

» Monitor for seizures

» Monitor for bleeding

Carotid Stenosis

Clinical presentation:

» TIAs, visual Δ's

» Memory loss

» Vertigo, syncope

» Carotid bruit or thrill

Treatment:

» Antiplatelet aggregation (ASA, Plavix)

» BP control

- Specific patient targets should be established

- Do not want to drop too much

» Balloon angioplasty (not done as much)

Carotid Endarterectomy:

» Post-op: Monitor for bleeding/hematoma

» Close airway monitoring (d/t location of incision)

» Neuro assessment

» Cranial nerve assessment:

- VII: Smile

- IX/X: Swallow, gag, speech

- XI: Shrug shoulders

- XII: Stick out tongue

Hemorrhagic Stroke

Causes:

» Spontaneous rupture
of a blood vessel

» Brain tumor bleed

» Uncontrolled anticoagulation

Who's at risk?

» Hypertension—the big one!

» Prior TIAs

» Diabetes

» Geriatric population

» Atrial fibrillation

» Trauma

» Smokers

Symptoms:

» Abrupt & rapid onset

» Hemiparesis

» Severe headache

» Posturing

» Nuchal rigidity

» Stupor, coma

**Severity depends on the size of the bleed

Treatment:

» Consider BP reduction if:

  * SBP > 200 or MAP > 150
  * More aggressive if increased
    ICPs & SBP > 180

» Airway support

» Monitor for seizures

» Nursing care same as
ischemic stroke

» Supportive treatment

Symptoms—all strokes

Right cerebral hemisphere:

» Left sided motor symptoms

» Respond well to verbal cues

» Can understand language

» Assists with cognition (thinking)

» Difficulty starting a conversation

» Rambling speech

» Issues with problem solving

Left cerebral hemisphere:

» Right sided motor symptoms

» Aphasia

» Expressive aphasia
  • Inability to express verbally in an understandable manner

» Receptive aphasia
  • Inability to understand spoken words

» Dyslexia

» Acalcia

» Right & left disorientation

» May respond well to pictures

» Memory loss

» Emotionally labile

Aneurysms

» Most occur in the anterior arteries of the Circle of Willis

» Rupture most likely when > 8 – 10 mm

» Congenital, vessel weakness or unknown

Risk factors:

- » Congenital

- » HTN

- » Smokers

- » Polycystic kidney disease
  (chronic hypertension)

Diagnosis:

- » CT Scan <u>WITHOUT</u> contrast

Symptoms:

- » Many are asymptomatic
  until they bleed/rupture

- » Symptoms & prognosis depend
  on the area & size of bleed

- » Sudden headache

- » "Worst headache of my life"

- » Nausea/vomiting

- » Photophobia

- » Diplopia

- » Nuchal rigidity

- » Kernig's sign and/or
  Brudzinski's sign

  * Indicates meningeal irritation

- » Seizures

- » Decreased LOC, may
  progress to coma

Treatment:

- » BP control

  * In general, keep SBP
    < 160 mm Hg

  * Needs to be patient specific target

- » Monitor for re-bleed

- » Days 4 – 14 monitor for
  cerebral artery vasospasm

  * Transcranial Doppler to monitor

  * High velocities
    indicative of spasm

  * Start prophylactic calcium
    channel blocker to prevent spasm

    ▷ Nimotop (Nimodipine) most
      commonly used

    ▷ Administered for about 1
      month

Post bleed/intervention, monitor for signs of:

» Increased ICP

» Cerebral edema

» Hydrocephalus

Interventions:

» Surgical & endovascular

» Bleed into subarachnoid space
  • CSF will be bloody

Arterial-Venous Malformation (AVM)

» Entanglement of blood vessels

» Concern with bleed or rupture

» Surgical and/or endovascular treatment

» Often congenital

Hydrocephalus

» Accumulation of CSF in the ventricles

Symptoms:

» Headache

» Decreased LOC, sleepy, confused

» Signs of increased ICP

» Seizures

Emergent treatment:

» Short term: Ventriculostomy

» Long term: VP Shunt

• Ventricle to pleural space or ventricle to peritoneal space

Seizures

» Abnormal electrical
  discharges in the brain

Causes:

» Genetic

» Congenital

» Exposure to drugs

» Withdrawal from
  drugs or alcohol

» Low sodium or glucose

» Infection

» Trauma

» Tumors

Duration can range from a few seconds to continuous without intervention

» 5 minutes is considered
  a medical emergency

Tonic-clonic (Grand mal) seizures:

Tonic phase:

» Lose consciousness

» Many times experience a fall

» Rigid extremities

» Bite tongue

» Pupils dilate

Clonic phase:

» Tachycardia

» Diaphoretic

» Frothing at mouth

» Violent, rhythmic shaking

» Alternating contraction
  & relaxation

Postictal phase:

» Altered LOC after seizure

» Lasts between 5 – 30 minutes, sometimes longer

» Drowsiness, confusion, hypertension, headache

Status Epilepticus

» Seizure lasts more than 30 min

» 20 – 30% mortality

» Safety is a priority!!!

  • Monitor for patent airway

  • Don't ever stick anything into the mouth!!!

» Identify the underlying cause

  • Consider toxicology screen

  • Assess electrolytes & glucose

Medications - Seizures

» Phenytoin (Dilantin)

  • Load 10 - 15 mg/kg or 15 - 20 mg/kg

  • Give slowly! 50 mg/min

  • Peak blood levels in 15 - 20 min

  • Monitor for bradycardia & hypotension

  • Assess levels; 10 – 20 mcg/L therapeutic level

  • Use a filter

  • Monitor IV site for infiltration

» Fosphenytoin

  • 150 mg/min

» Valproic acid

» Benzodiazepines

  • Lorazepam

  • Diazepam

Guillain-Barré Syndrome

» Autoimmune disorder

» Immune system attacks the peripheral nervous system

» Many times follows when recovering from an illness or virus

» Usually 1 - 3 weeks after

» Temporary damage to the myelin sheath

» Impulses travel slow causing slow movements or paralysis

» Peak incidence age 30 - 40

Symptoms:

» Paresthesia (numbness & tingling)

» Pins & needles hands, feet & face

» Uncoordinated movements

» Blurred vision
  * Unilateral or bilateral

» Loss of DTRs/areflexia

» Difficulty breathing

» Muscle weakness usually starts in legs, then arms, face & respiratory

» Ascending paralysis

Diagnosis:

» Lumbar puncture

» Albuminocytologic dissociation in the CSF

» High protein level, few cells

Treatment options:

» Plasmapheresis

» IVIG (immunoglobulin)

» It is not understood why either treatment works

Supportive treatment:

» DVT prophylaxis

» Nutritional support

» Physical Therapy

» Neurogenic bowel & bladder

» Prevent infections!!!

» Psychosocial support

» Airway, monitor for respiratory failure
  * ~ 30% require mechanical ventilation

» Recovery weeks to months

Meningitis

» Inflammation of the meninges

Symptoms:

» Headache

» Nuchal rigidity

» Fever

» Altered LOC

» Photophobia, phonophobia

» + Brudzinski's sign

* Severe neck stiffness causes a patient's hips and knees to flex when the neck is flexed

» + Kernig's sign

* Severe stiffness of the hamstrings causes an inability to straighten the leg when the hip is flexed to 90 degrees

Diagnosis:

» Lumbar puncture

» If it's viral meningitis, the results will show:

* + Protein in CSF

* Normal glucose in CSF

* Lymphocytes

* Enteroviruses, herpes simplex virus, varicella zoster virus, HIV

» If it's bacterial meningitis, the results will show:

* +++ Protein in CSF

* Low glucose in CSF

* Neutrophils, WBCs

* Rash may indicate meningococcal infection

* Neisseria meningitis & streptococcus pneumoniae 80% of cases

Lumbar puncture FYIs:

» Usually L4 – L5 interspace

» Assess "opening pressure", normal: 6 – 18 mm Hg

CSF sample to assess:

» WBC, RBC, Protein, glucose, gram stain

  * CSF glucose is usually 40% higher than serum

  * Bacterial meningitis—divide CSF glucose by serum glucose

    ▷ Index ≤ 0.4

  * Assess for lactate (Increased level = Bacterial)

» Supine position post LP

Hypoxic-Ischemic Brain Injury

» aka "anoxic injury"

» Loss of distinction between gray & white matter in the cerebral hemispheres

» Happens after cardiac or respiratory arrests & drownings

» Global brain ischemia caused from cessation of cerebral blood flow

» Major injury happens during reperfusion

Treatment:

» Targeted temperature management to minimize reperfusion injury

What happens during arrest & reperfusion?

» Depleted stores of O_2 & glucose

» Intracellular calcium influx

» Formation of O_2 free radicals

» Release of glutamate

» Intracellular acidosis

» Disruption in blood brain barrier

» Mitochondrial injury

» Apoptosis

Targeted Temperature Management:

» Only in patients remaining comatose post cardiac arrest

» Reason: neuro protection

» 32 – 36 degrees C for 24 hours

» Slow re-warming back to normal temperature

» Avoid fevers post cardiac arrest

Side effects of cooling: (seen when cooled to 32 – 34 degree range)

» Bradycardia

» Vasoconstriction induced hypertension

» Diuresis

» Hypokalemia—d/t electrolyte shifting

» Elevated lactate

» Insulin resistance

» Mild coagulopathy

» Shivering—observed at all temperature ranges

Re-warming:

» Should be done very slowly

» 0.15 – 0.25° C per hour

You can do it!

Pulmonary Review

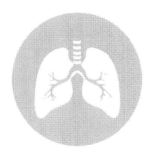

AACN Blueprint for the Pulmonary portion of the CCRN® Exam

- Acute pulmonary embolus

- Acute respiratory distress syndrome (ARDS), acute lung injury (ALI) & respiratory distress syndrome (RDS)

- Acute respiratory failure

- Acute respiratory infections

- Air-leak syndromes

- Aspiration

- Chronic conditions—COPD, Asthma, Bronchitis, emphysema

- Failure to wean from the ventilator

- Pulmonary fibrosis

- Pulmonary hypertension

- Status Asthmaticus

- Thoracic surgery

- Thoracic Trauma (fractured rib, lung contusion, tracheal perforation)

General Assessment

» Crackles (rales)—heart failure, effusions, pneumonia

» Rhonchi (coarse)—Secretions in large airways, pneumonia

» Wheezes—narrowed airways (note if inspiration / expiration)

Arterial Blood Gases

Know the norms!

Normal blood gas values:

pH:	7.35 – 7.45
PaO$_2$:	80 – 100
PaCO$_2$:	35 – 45
HCO$_3$:	22 – 26
Base Deficit:	-2 to +2
SaO$_2$:	95 – 100%

Lungs: Fast compensation

Kidneys: Slow compensation

If the pH is < 7.35, that leans toward acidosis, > 7.45 leans toward alkalosis

If the PaCO$_2$ is < 35, that leans toward alkalosis, > 45 leans toward acidosis

If the HCO$_3$ is < 22, that leans toward acidosis, > 26 leans toward alkalosis

Be methodical when interpreting ABGs

» Look at 3 main values to interpret: pH, PaCO$_2$, HCO$_3$...hold that thought!

Easy method for ABG interpretation:

» Every ABG will have a first name, middle name & last name

Example: pH = 7.31, $PaCO_2$ = 54, PaO_2 = 97, HCO_3 = 24

» First name: assess the pH

* Is it normal or abnormal?

  ▷ 7.31 = abnormal

  ▷ Abnormal = <u>Uncompensated</u>

» Last name: assess the pH again

* Is it leaning toward acidosis or alkalosis?

  ▷ 7.31 = <u>Acidosis</u>

» Middle name: assess the $PaCO_2$ & HCO_3

* Which one is leaning toward acidosis?

  ▷ The $PaCO_2$ is! (<u>Respiratory</u>)

* If the $PaCO_2$ is the cause the middle name will be respiratory

* If the HCO_3 was the cause, the middle name would be metabolic

» Interpretation: <u>uncompensated respiratory acidosis</u>

Another tip...

» Look at the pH & CO_2

If the pH & CO_2 are both up or both down:

* sa**ME** = **Me**tabolic

Example: pH 7.32 (↓) CO_2: 32 (↓) HCO_3: 18

* **Re**verse = **Re**spiratory

Example: pH: 7.28 (↓) CO_2: 54 (↑) HCO_3: 26

ROME—<u>R</u>espiratory <u>O</u>pposite, <u>M</u>etabolic <u>E</u>qual

» Examples:

* pH 7.36 $PaCO_2$ 48 HCO_3 24
  Compensated Respiratory Acidosis

* pH 7.26 $PaCO_2$ 35 HCO_3 16
  Uncompensated Metabolic Acidosis (pH & HCO_3 lean toward acid)

160 Pulmonary Review

* pH 7.30 $PaCO_2$ 58 HCO_3 30
Partially Compensated Respiratory Acidosis (pH & $PaCo_2$ lean toward acid, HCO_3 is leaning in opposite direction; change 1st name to partially compensated)

» Respiratory Acidosis Example

* pH 7.22 $PaCO_2$ 65 HCO_3 24
Uncompensated Respiratory Acidosis

» Respiratory Acidosis Causes:

* Over-sedation
* Late respiratory failure
* Drug overdoses that cause respiratory depression
* COPD
* Brain stem dysfunction
* Extreme V/Q mismatch, Pulmonary embolus, PNA
* Guillain Barré Syndrome
* Excessive CO_2 production (Sepsis, TPN, burns)
* Think hypoventilation! (retaining CO_2)

» Respiratory Alkalosis Example:

* pH 7.52 $PaCO_2$ 26 HCO_3 22
Uncompensated Respiratory Alkalosis

» Respiratory Alkalosis Causes:

* Early respiratory failure
* Anxiety or severe pain
* Excessive tidal volume or rate on ventilator
* ARDs
* Heart failure
* Neurologic disorders
* Pulmonary embolus
* Salicylate overdose (adults)
* Decreased cardiac output/shock
* PaO_2 < 60 (cause & effect)
* Think hyperventilation! (blowing off CO_2)

» Metabolic Acidosis Example:

* pH 7.16 $PaCO_2$ 35 HCO_3 14
Uncompensated Metabolic Acidosis

» Metabolic Acidosis Causes:

* Acute kidney injury

* Drug overdoses

* Diabetic ketoacidosis

* Sepsis

* Lactic acidosis

* Toxins

* Aspirin overdose

* Liver failure

* Hyperkalemia, hyperchloremia

» Calculate an anion gap!!!

* **Anion gap: normal < 11 – 12**

  ▷ > 12—associated with metabolic acidosis

* Easy acronym for common metabolic acidosis:

M: Methanol

U: Uremia

D: DKA

P: Propylene glycol

I: Isoniazid

L: Lactic Acidosis

E: Ethylene glycol

S: Salicylates

» Metabolic Alkalosis Example:

* pH 7.49 $PaCO_2$ 36 HCO_3 29
  Uncompensated Metabolic Alkalosis

» Metabolic Alkalosis Causes:

* NG tube to suction

* Emesis

* Hypokalemia

* Hypochloremia

* Antacid abuse

* Excessive sodium bicarb infusion

* Inadequate renal perfusion

* Diuretics

* Excessive albuterol use

* Hyperaldosteronism (d/t RAAS activation)

Hypoxemia

Three main reasons:

» Hypoventilation

- ↓ Total volume air inhaled/exhaled
- ↓ Phosphate or magnesium levels
- Obstructive sleep apnea

» Ventilation/perfusion (V/Q) mismatch

- PE, pneumonia, shunt

» DO_2/VO_2 imbalance

- ↓ Cardiac output
- Severe anemia

Intrapulmonary Shunt

» V/Q mismatch

» Excessive blood flow in relation to ventilation

» Ventilation without perfusion (pulmonary embolism)

Examples of shunting:

» Asthma—small airways restricted

» Pulmonary edema— alveoli filled with fluid

» Atelectasis—alveolar collapse

» Pulmonary embolus—non-embolized regions of the lungs (lots of deadspace!)

» PaO_2 decreases as shunt increases

» In general, $PaCO_2$ stays about the same

Oxygen

» Too much is NOT a good thing!

» Too little is also NOT a good thing!

» O_2 is a vasoconstrictor in all vascular beds except the lungs (vasodilator)

» Extensive oxygen has negative inotropic effects on the heart

Delivery Methods

» Nasal cannula 1 - 6 L

  * 21% to 46% FiO_2

  * High flow cannula

» Face Mask 5 - 10 L

  * 40% to 60% FiO_2

» Partial re-breather mask 5 - 7 L

  * 35% to 75% FiO_2

» Non-rebreather mask 5 - 10 L

  * 40% to 100% FiO_2

Asthma

Characteristics:

» Airway hyperactivity

» Inflammation

» Bronchial constriction

» Excessive mucus production

» Air trapping with hyperinflation of the lungs

» Lots of resistance!

» Can air trap causing AUTO-PEEP

  * Increased pressure in distal airways

Treatment:

» 1st Line Therapy: BRONCHODILATORS!!!!

» aka - Beta$_2$ agonist

» Albuterol—onset < 5 min

  * Effects last 2 - 5 hours

  * Repetitive or continuous albuterol nebs:

  * 2.5 mg per treatment

  * Continuous: 5 - 15 mg/hr

Side effects of Albuterol:

» Tachycardia

» Tremors (stimulates Beta$_2$ receptors)

» Hyperglycemia

» Hypomagnesemia

» Hypokalemia

» Hypophosphatemia

Other asthma treatments:

Anticholinergic Agents

» Ipratropium bromide (Atrovent)

» Derivative of atropine

» Only in combination with Beta$_2$ agonist (like albuterol)

» Conflicting evidence

» Used in severe exacerbation

» 0.5 mg neb every 20 min x 3, then every 2 – 4 hours

» MDI 4 – 8 puffs

Corticosteroids

» Reduces secondary airway inflammation & edema

» Prevents relapse

» Methylprednisolone or prednisone for 7 – 10 days

» Neither PO or IV is superior, benefit not seen until 12 hours after therapy started

» No need to taper

» Monitor for myopathies

Other thoughts on asthma treatment:

» No O$_2$ unless ↓ O$_2$ sats

» No CXR unless suspect PNA

» No ABG unless non-responsive to therapy

» No antibiotics unless there is an infection!

» Hypercapnia is an ominous sign

» Can consider Magnesium Sulfate 1 - 2 grams over 2 hours

• Bronchodilation effects

» Heliox (helium & oxygen combination)

• Decreases resistance in airways

If need for mechanical ventilation:

» Lower ventilation rate (allows more time in exhalation)

» Prolonged expiratory pause

» Decrease minute ventilation

» Lower tidal volume

» Monitor for auto-PEEP

Chronic Obstructive Pulmonary Disease (COPD)

» Umbrella term for emphysema & chronic bronchitis

» Constant airflow obstruction

» Worsens over time

» Diagnosis: Pulmonary Function Test

  * $FEV_1/FVC < 70\%$
  * Normal: 80%

» Shortness of breath

» Cough, +/- Sputum

Other characteristics of COPD—Emphysema

» Air-trapping with chronic hyperinflation of lungs

» Prolonged exhalation

» Barrel chest

» Clubbed fingers

» Enlarged right heart

» Elevated right sided venous pressures (CVP)

» Develop intrinsic PEEP from air trapping

COPD Exacerbation Treatment:

» Bronchodilators—some thought there may be limited benefit

» Short course of corticosteroids—7 to 10 days

  * Methylprednisolone or prednisone

  * No advantage of IV over PO

  * Inhaled steroids longterm and bronchodilators

» Antibiotics are debated as many infections are viral

  * Strep pneumonia

* H. flu
* Problem: antibiotic resistance

» Oxygen therapy general guideline:

* Keep O_2 sats low 90% range, avoid high concentration of O_2
* If O_2 needed, monitor for signs of hypercapnia

» Non-invasive ventilation

* CPAP for hypoxic failure

* Bi-Pap for hypercapnic failure

» Intubate if:

* Respiratory distress with hemodynamic compromise
* Mental status change, somnolence
* Worsening acidosis
* Monitor for intrinsic PEEP (Auto-PEEP)
  ▷ Increased pressure in distal airways

COPD vs. Asthma

» COPD

* Onset in mid-life
* Symptoms slowly progressive
* Long smoking history

» Asthma

* Onset early in life (often childhood)
* Symptoms vary from day to day
* Symptoms worse at night/ early morning
* Allergy, rhinitis, and/or eczema also present
* Family history of asthma

Acute Respiratory Failure

Oxygen or ventilation disturbance

Q > V (Perfusion exceeds ventilation)

Signs:

» Increased work of breathing

» Use of accessory muscles

» Increased minute ventilation

* Compensating for: increased dead space

» Hallmark sign of <u>late</u> failure:

* Increased $PaCO_2$/Hypercapnia!!!

Who is at risk? (Many patients!)

» COPD

» Pneumonia

» Pulmonary edema

» ARDS

» Drug overdoses

» Restrictive lung disease

Non-Invasive Ventilation (NPPV)

CPAP/BiPAP

» Continuous positive pressure

» Stabilizes airways during exhalation

» Improves ventilation

» Keeps alveoli open

» Used to treat:
  * COPD Exacerbation
  * CHF, pulmonary edema
  * Obstructive sleep apnea
  * Obesity hypoventilation syndrome

CPAP

» Simple mask & O_2

» Set at 5 – 10 cm H_2O

» Increases functional residual capacity

» Does not augment tidal volume

Bi-PAP

» Bi-level positive airway pressure

» CPAP that alternates between 2 pressure levels

» Higher mean airway pressures, more alveolar recruitment

» Provides larger tidal volumes

» Set IPAP & EPAP

» Typical starting point:
  * IPAP 10 cm H_2O, EPAP 5 cm H_2O
  * Inspiratory time 3 seconds

Acute Respiratory Distress Syndrome (ARDS)

» Inflammatory lung disease

» It is not a primary disease, but a result of:

* Sepsis

* Trauma

* Multiple blood transfusions (TRALI, CRALI)

* Pancreatitis

* Cardiopulmonary bypass

* Pulmonary contusion

* Pneumonia/aspiration

What is happening in ARDS?

» INFLAMMATORY RESPONSE!

» Alveoli are infiltrated with leukocytes

» Fibrin deposits in lungs

» Widespread endothelial & alveolar damage

» Leaky capillaries

» Lungs get stiff

» Decreased compliance

» Non-cardiogenic pulmonary edema

Signs:

» Tachypnea

» Progressive refractory hypoxemia

» Worsening P/F ratio

* (PaO$_2$ divided by FiO$_2$)

» CXR—Bilateral pulmonary infiltrates

» Usually require mechanical ventilation within 48 hours

» What therapy will improve the PaO$_2$?

* Answer: PEEP!

Diagnosis:

» Pulmonary infiltrates on CXR

» P/F ratio: PaO$_2$ ÷ FiO$_2$

Berlin Criteria—2012

» P/F ratio:

  * < 300—Mild ARDS

  * < 200—Moderate ARDS

  * < 100—Severe ARDS

» Predisposing conditions

» Absence of left heart failure or left atrial hypertension

» Mimics pneumonia & cardiogenic pulmonary edema

» Broncho-alveolar Lavage (BAL) or Bronchoscopy

  * Sample examined for neutrophils & protein

  * Neutrophils: Up to 80% in ARDS

    ▷ Normal: 5%

  * Higher protein level in aspirate, sign of inflammation

ARDS Treatment:

» Mechanical ventilation with "Lung Protective Ventilation" or "LPV"

» Low tidal volumes; goal 6 ml/kg

» Larger tidal volumes over distend & rupture distal air space (volutrauma)

» Limit pressure related injury (barotrauma)

» Use predicted body weight when establishing tidal volume settings

» Goal: End inspiratory plateau pressure < 30 cm H_2O

  * Inspiratory hold on the ventilator—measure pressure at that point

» Allow permissive hypercapnia

» Use of PEEP

  * Think of PEEP as a stent to keep alveoli open

» When increasing PEEP, monitor for signs of decreased cardiac output!!!

  * May see hypotension

» Use Neuromuscular blockade if dysynchrony with the ventilator

  * Peripheral nerve stimulation ("train of four") to monitor dosing

  * Goal: 1 – 2 twitches out of 4 electrical stimuli

  * Advantages of NM Blockade:

    ▷ Decreases barotrauma

    ▷ Decreases ventilator days

    ▷ Decreases pro-inflammatory response

Other therapies:

» Conservative fluid management

  * Diuretics

  * Do NOT fluid overload patients!

  * Able to liberate the patient from the ventilator quicker!

» Optimize O_2 delivery

  * Cardiac Output: Dobutamine

  * PaO_2: PEEP

  * Low hemoglobin: Transfuse only if necessary!

» Steroids

  * No benefit from early steroids

  * Some benefit days 7 – 14

  * Methylprednisolone 2 – 3 mg/kg/day

  * Inhibits fibrinolysis

» Prone positioning

  * New evidence of benefit

  * Must be done <u>early</u>, not used as a last ditch treatment

  * Should remain prone > 16 hours per day

Capnography—PEtCO$_2$

» Is a measure of ventilation, but also a reflection of perfusion & metabolism

  * If cardiac output drops, capnography values will drop

» Continuous with waveform

» Normal Capnography is 35 – 45 mm Hg

» PEtCO$_2$ should be within 5 mm Hg of PaCO$_2$

» Is the gold standard way to verify endotracheal tube placement

  * Lungs vs. gut...still need a chest x-ray to determine how high or low ET tube is

» Standard of care for moderate to deep sedation

» Helpful to calculate deadspace & V/Q matching in certain conditions, like:

  * Pulmonary embolus

  * Pneumonia

  * Over-distention of alveoli from PEEP or tidal volume

  * Endotracheal tube in main stem bronchus

  * Asthma or COPD exacerbation

» As a measure of perfusion, capnography is helpful with:

* Resuscitation (CPR quality & ROSC)

* Low cardiac output states = low $PEtCO_2$

* Correlation between $PEtCO_2$ & Cardiac Output

» Other uses:

* Weaning the ventilator

* Head injuries

* Used with PCAs/sedating agents

Pulmonary Embolus

» 70% have a DVT

Signs:

» Tachycardia

» Tachypnea

» Dyspnea

» Chest pain

» Hemoptysis

» Sudden right heart failure

» Increased PA pressures

» PEA Arrest

Diagnosis

» Spiral (helical) CT scan— detector rotated around the patient; 2-D view

* 30 seconds to do scan

* Ideal hold breath for 30 seconds!

* Contrast infused to view pulmonary vasculature

* 93% sensitivity / 97% specificity if clot is in one of the main arteries

Other diagnostics:

» Pulmonary angiogram

* Most accurate

* Performed in < 20% of patients with PE because it takes too long

» Ultrasound—DVT extremities

» V/Q Scan—only diagnoses 25 – 30% of cases

- Underlying lung disease—abnormal scan

» 12 Lead ECG findings:

  - Right axis deviation
  - Transient right BBB

- ST depression, T wave depression in $V_1 - V_4$

» Tall peaked T waves in II, III, aVF

» ABG—low PaO_2

Treatment:

If hemodynamically stable:

» Unfractionated Heparin (UFH)

  - Weight-based dosing
  - Prevent progression
  - Bolus, then continuous infusion
  - Goal: aPTT 50 – 80 seconds

» Warfarin

  - Used with UFH
  - Usually start on 1st day of Heparin therapy
  - Goal: INR 2 – 3, then d/c Heparin
  - Continue for 6 weeks

Can also use:

» Low Molecular Weight Heparin (LMWH)

» Enoxaparin 1 mg/kg Q 12 hours

  - Cleared by the kidneys (renal adjustment)
  - Simplified dosing
  - No need to monitor coags
  - Treat outpatient

If the patient has hemodynamic instability or cardiac arrest:

» Fibrinolytic therapy

  - Alteplase—0.6 mg/kg over 15 min or
  - Reteplase—10 unit IV bolus, repeat in 30 min
  - 12% chance of major hemorrhage

  - 1% ICH
  - Have to weigh benefit > risk

IVC Filters

Used for DVT if:

» Contraindication to
anticoagulation

» Pulmonary embolus while
on anticoagulation

» Thrombus in right heart
or free floating

Pulmonary Arterial Hypertension (PAH)

» High pressure in the
pulmonary vasculature

» Leads to right sided heart failure

Causes:

» Idiopathic

» Medications

» Systemic hypertension

» Obstructive sleep apnea (OSA)

» Sclerotic diseases

Common treatments for symptomatic PAH (oral):

» Sildenafil (Viagra)

» Bosentan (Tracleer)

Rapid progression treatment:

» Epoprostenol (Flolan)—
Continuous IV (short half-life)

- Always have an extra
  bag on standby

» Treprostinil (Remodulin)

» Goal with all meds is
pulmonary vasodilation

» Watch for hypotension

Pulmonary Contusion

Mechanism of Injury

» Damage to the parenchyma of the lung

» Localized edema

» Hemorrhage, rupture capillaries

Symptoms:

» Not always immediate—24 to 72 hours, once swelling starts!

» Tachypnea

» Tachycardia

» Hypoxemia

» Hemoptysis—pink, frothy

» Crackles

» External signs of ecchymosis, rib fractures

Diagnosis:

» CT scan—most sensitive

» Differentiate between atelectasis & aspiration

» ↓ P/F ratio

» ↓ $PaCO_2$ (d/t ↑ RR)
  • Early failure—blow off CO_2

Treatment:

» Supportive with severe contusions, treat like ARDS

» Do not fluid overload!!!

Rib fractures

» 4 - 8 most common

» 9 - 12 concern with rupture of spleen, liver or diaphragmatic tear

» Diagnosed by chest x-ray

» Pain control—consider epidural catheter

» **Prevent Pneumonia
  • Encourage incentive spirometer

Hemothorax

» Blood in the pleural space

* Lung tissue is compressed, collapses alveoli

* Often accompanied by a pneumothorax

Causes:

» Trauma, thoracic surgery, thoracic aneurysm

» > 400 mls—symptomatic

» Hypovolemia & shock

» Respiratory acidosis, dropping hemoglobin

» Absent breath sounds on affected side

» CT scan to diagnose

» Place chest tube

» Thoracotomy if unable to control bleeding

Pneumothorax

» Air in the pleural space

Causes:

» Trauma

» Too much PEEP

» Ruptured bleb

» Lung disease (COPD, cystic fibrosis, pneumonia)

3 types:

» Closed

* Air enters through airways & cannot escape

* ↑ Intrathoracic chest pressure

* ↑ Pressure on lungs & heart → leads to tension pneumothorax

» Tension (the really bad one!)

- Life threatening
- Air accumulates in pleural space & cannot escape
- Pressure collapses the lung
- Decreased capacity, decreased compliance

- Can lead to PEA Arrest

» Open

- Penetrating injury
- Air enters & exits
- Less dangerous

Signs & Symptoms:

» Depends on size

» Dyspnea

» Restlessness

» Anxiety

» Chest pain

» SOB

» Cyanosis

» Decreased or absent breath sounds on affected side

» Tracheal shift toward unaffected side

Treatment:

» Diagnosed by chest x-ray

» ABG—low PaO_2

» If it is small, treatment may not be necessary

- (air will be reabsorbed)

» If larger pneumo, chest tube

» Emergent needle decompression:

- 14 – 16 gauge needle
- 2nd ICS, midclavicular line, right above 3rd rib
- Listen for air escaping

Chest Tubes:

» Use suction to re-expand the lung

» 10 – 20 cm H_2O suction (or up to 40 cm H_2O suction with dry suction)

» Bubbling in water seal is normal with pneumothorax

* Otherwise not normal & need to trouble shoot reason for leak

* Or, a possible new pneumo!

» When bubbling stops, air evacuated from pleural space

» Do NOT clamp chest tubes if bubbling in H_2O seal chamber!!!

» Follow CXR

» Do NOT milk or strip chest tubes…it can create up to -400 cm H_2O pressure!!!

Advanced airways

Endotracheal Tubes

» Nasal or oral

» Smaller number = smaller tube

» Placement confirmed via waveform Capnography**

* Auscultate chest (not overly helpful)

* Chest x-ray done to verify placement

* ET tube should sit 2 – 3 cm above carina

» Ideal cuff pressure 20 – 30 cm H_2O

Tracheostomy Tubes

» Used if long term support anticipated

» Emergency—obstruction

» Always have an extra trach at the patient's bedside

» Keep clean—avoid hydrogen peroxide

» Can deflate the cuff so the patient can talk

* Use a one-way valve

Mechanical ventilation

Basic settings:

» Mode of ventilation

* Ventilator brand dependent, but usually pressure or volume or a combo of both

» Rate (breaths per minute)

» Tidal volume

* Volume of air in/out of lungs

* Based on <u>predicted body weight</u>—if you gain weight your lung size doesn't change!

* PBW Chart—gender and height

» PEEP

» FiO_2

Modes of ventilation—volume

AMV—Assisted Mandatory Ventilation

» Also called assist control

» Preset tidal volume & minimum rate of breaths

» Able to initiate breaths, but will get set tidal volume

» Patient can alter rate & pattern, but not the tidal volume

» Reduces work of breathing

SIMV—Synchronized Intermittent Mandatory Ventilation

» Preset rate & tidal volume

» Allows patient to spontaneously breathe in between breaths

» Synchronized with patient initiated breath

» Reduces competition between patent & ventilator

» High set rate allows no time for the patient to spontaneously breath

» Can use IMV + pressure support

Modes of ventilation—pressure

PCV—Pressure Control Ventilation

» Set inflation pressure

» Inspiratory time adjusted to allow time for inspiratory flow rate to drop to zero at end inspiration

PS—Pressure Support

» Delivery of positive pressure

» Patient decides when, how fast & flow

» Assistance during inspiration; must initiate breath

» Set back up apnea mode

» Ideal pressure support to achieve Vt 6 – 8 ml/kg

» Used for weaning

Combo modes of ventilation:

VC—Volume Control

» Also called PRVC—Pressure Regulated Volume Control

» Pressure controlled breaths

» Guaranteed minimum volume

» Ventilator adjusts pressure & flow to achieve minimum Vt

APRV—Airway Pressure Release Ventilation

» Cycles between high & low continuous positive airway pressure

» P high—delivered for a longer period of time

» P low—for shorter time

» Transition between high/ low deflates the lungs and allows for CO_2 removal

» Time spent in P high determines the rate

Weaning (now called "liberation" from the ventilator)

» Determine readiness

» Spontaneous breathing trial (SBT)

» Lighten sedation/analgesia

* Spontaneous awakening trial (SAT)

* SBTs should ALWAYS be paired with SATs

* Patient must be awake!

When weaning, assess:

» Vital capacity

* Highest volume of air exhaled with the deepest effort of breath

» RR during weaning

» NIF—Negative Inspiratory Force

» PIP—Peak Inspiratory Effort

» NIF & PIP of - 20 cm H_2O good sign for extubation

* Normal is: – 70 to – 90

» Nutrition—Phosphate levels should be adequate

Breathing trials in general:

» Should last < 2 hours

» CPAP or pressure support

» Decrease rate

» T-piece

» Monitor oximetry & $PEtCO_2$

* If the $PEtCO_2$ increases during the trial, patient is likely not ready to liberate

* Increasing $PEtCO_2$ is a sign of ineffective ventilation

» Monitor minute ventilation

* Amount of air exchanged in 1 minute

* Normal is 5 – 10 L/min

Contraindications to extubation:

» Absence of gag reflex

» Unable to protect airway

» Absence of cuff leak (edema)

Post-extubation:

» Monitor for stridor

» Hypercapnia

Ventilator Associated Events (VAE, aka VAP prevention):

» HOB elevation (30 – 45 degrees)

» Mouth/endotracheal tube care (oral w/chlorhexidine)

» Lung Protective Ventilator Strategies

» Early discontinuation of ventilator

» Daily interruption of sedation

» Appropriate analgesia & sedation (avoid benzos)

» Early mobilization with or without ambulation

» DVT Prophylaxis

» GI Prophylaxis (use cautiously in appropriate patients!)

» Balanced IV fluid administration

You can do it!

Renal, Genitourinary & Electrolytes Review

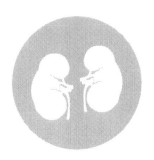

AACN Blueprint for the Renal, GU & Electrolyte portion of the CCRN® Exam:

- Acute kidney injury (AKI)
- Acute renal failure
- Acute tubular necrosis (ATN)
- Chronic kidney disease
- Incontinence
- Infections
- Life threatening electrolyte imbalances

Overview of the renal system

» Approximately 20% of cardiac output goes to the kidneys

» Renal arteries branch directly off aorta

Main function of the kidneys

» Cleanse & detoxify blood

» Filtration

» Reabsorption of water electrolytes, amino acids

» Secretion of water & wastes

» Acid/base balance

» Blood pressure regulation

» Erythropoietin production

The nephron is made of the:

» **Glomerulus**

  * Network of capillaries

  * Filters blood

» **Proximal Convoluted Tubule**

  * Reabsorbs H_2O, sodium, amino acids & glucose

» **Loop of Henle**

  * Reabsorbs Na^+, water & concentrates urine

  * This is where loop diuretics work (i.e. Lasix)

» **Distal Convoluted Tubule**

  * Regulates pH, K^+, Na^+ & Ca^{++}

» **Collecting Duct**

  * Collects urine from the nephrons

Fluid balance is regulated by:

» Thirst

» Anti-diuretic hormone (ADH)

» Aldosterone

» Elevated K^+ triggers release of aldosterone

» Atria-natriuretic peptide (ANP)

  * Overstretch of the atria triggers the kidneys to hold on to water

» Renin Angiotensin Aldosterone System (RAAS)

  * When activated, triggers the kidneys to hold onto sodium & water

Urine

» **Normal urine output**

* 1 – 1.5 L/day or 0.5 mL/kg/hour

» **Anuria**

* < 100 mL/day

» **Oliguria**

* < 400 mL/day

» **Polyuria**

* > 2500 mL/day

Acute Kidney Injury (AKI)

» a.k.a. Acute renal failure (ARF)

» Abrupt decline in glomerular filtration rate (GFR)

» Results in retention of metabolic waste

* Protein catabolism (azotemia)

* Electrolyte & acid-base imbalance (retention of potassium, magnesium & phosphate, acidosis)

* Fluid overload

Causes of acute kidney injury:

» Low perfusion, medications, parenchymal disease

» Reversible if prompt treatment is received

Risk factors for developing AKI

» Elderly

» Heart failure

» Baseline renal function

» Elevated body mass index (BMI > 32)

» COPD

» Liver disease

» Sepsis

» GI Bleeding

» Burns & trauma

» Multi-System Organ Failure

» Hypotension/decreased C.O.

» Rhabdomyolysis

» Contrast dye

» Hypovolemia for whatever reason

Labs to assess in AKI

» Azotemia—elevated BUN

» Elevated creatinine

  • Up to 12 hour lag time in elevation. Not an early indicator!

» BUN/Creatinine ratio, normal ratio is 10:1

» Glomerular Filtration Rate (estimated by creatinine clearance)

» Urinalysis:

  • Casts - presence is a sign of tubular cell death

  • Electrolytes (specifically Na^+)

  • Albumin

  • Glucose

  • Protein

Glomerular Filtration Rate (GFR)

» Estimated by assessing *creatinine clearance*

» The measurement of how much filtrate is made by the kidney (ml/min)

» Normal creatinine clearance is about 80 – 120 ml/min

» It is used to evaluate the kidneys' ability to remove waste products from the body

» Males have a creatinine clearance slightly higher than females

» Isolated plasma creatinine is not a sensitive marker for GFR in early stages of kidney injury

Equations used to estimate GFR (this is FYI only!)

» Cockcroft-Gault

$$GFR = (140 - age) \times (weight) / (sCr \times 72) \ (\times 0.85 \text{ for } ♀)$$

OR

» MDRD—Modification of Diet in Renal Disease

$$GFR = 186 \times (serum\ creatinine\ in\ mg/dL)^{-1.154}$$
$$\times (Age\ in\ years) - 0.203 \ (\times 0.742\ if\ female)$$
$$(\times 1.210\ if\ African\text{-}American)$$

Acute Kidney Injury (AKI)

Three Categories of AKI:

Postrenal AKI

» Think obstruction!

» Injury caused by disruption of urine flow

» Causes: urethral obstruction, prostate disease, infection, neurogenic bladder (i.e. spinal cord injury), blood clots, stones

» Oliguria

» Normal BUN/Creatinine ratio 10 - 15:1 (but, both elevated!)

» Creatinine > 1.2 mg/dL

» Urine specific gravity < 1.01, urine osmo < 350, urine Na^+ > 40 mEq/L

Treatment:

» Remove obstruction

» Will likely need bladder catheter

Prerenal AKI

» Results from hypoperfusion

» Kidney structure & function is preserved

» Causes: Sepsis, heart failure, trauma, severe hypovolemia

» BUN/Creatinine ratio > 20:1 (BUN elevates, creatinine may start to elevate)

» Oliguria

» Urine Na^+ < 20 mEq/L (kidneys hold on to Na^+ & H_2O)

» Urine osmo & urine specific gravity ↑ due to concentration

» HIGH RISK for progressing to ATN!

Treatment:

» Treat cause, improve perfusion

Acute Tubular Necrosis (ATN)

» May also be referred to "intrarenal" kidney injury

» Injury occurs at the nephron; there is structural damage!

» Causes: Hypotension, glomerulonephritis, diabetes, rhabdomyolysis, nephrotoxic medications, shock states

» BUN/Creatinine ratio 10:1 (Both BUN & creatinine are elevated)

» BUN > 25 mg/dL, creatinine > 1.2 mg/dL

» Often requires renal replacement therapy (RRT)/dialysis

Treatment:

» Depends on cause, assess if dialysis is indicated

» Prevent acidosis, electrolyte imbalance & uremia

» Stop nephrotoxic medications

» Ensure adequate cardiac output

Two types of Acute Tubular Necrosis (ATN):

Ischemic ATN

» Irregular damage along tubular membranes

» Tubular cell damage & cast formation

» Poor perfusion to kidneys

» Recovery long (> 8 days)

Toxic ATN

» Caused by drugs or bacteria

» Aminoglycosides & antivirals are common offenders

» Uniform, wide spread damage to the renal tubules

» Recovery more rapid (< 8 days)

» ***Reversible if offending cause is stopped!

Three distinct phases of ATN:

Oliguric Phase

» Insult to injury within 48 hours

» Inability to excrete fluids
& metabolic wastes

» Significant increase in
BUN & creatinine

» Fluid overload, acidosis

» Electrolyte imbalance
(especially K^+)

» Urine Na^+ < 10 mEq/L

» Often requires dialysis

Diuretic Phase

» Lasts 7 – 14 days

» Gradual improvement
in renal function

» Increase in GFR & often
develop polyuria

» Urine output 2 – 5 L/day

» Hemodialysis may cover polyuria

» Kidneys can often clear volume,
but not solute or waste

» Waste electrolyte—monitor
K^+ & Na^+ closely!

» Urine specific gravity <
1.01, urine osmo < 350,
urine Na^+ > 20 - 40

» Monitor for fluid deficit

Recovery Phase

» Can progress to CKD

» GFR returns to < 80% of
normal within 1 – 2 years

Summary of each type of failure:

	Prerenal	(ATN) Intrarenal	Postrenal
Urine Volume	Oliguria	Oliguria in Oliguric phase, polyuria in diuretic phase	Oliguric to anuria
Specific Gravity (normal 1.01 – 1.02)	>1.02	↑in oliguric phase, ↓in diuretic phase	Normal to elevated
Urinary Sodium (normal 40 – 100)	< 20 mEq/L	< 10 mEq/L in oliguric phase, > 20 - 40 mEq/L in diuretic phase	> 40 mEq/L
Urinary Sediment	Normal No protein	Erythrocyte and/or tubular casts, hematuria Proteinuria	Possible bacteria
BUN to Creatinine ratio (normal 10:1)	> 20:1	10:1 – 15:1 (both elevated)	10:1 – 15:1 (both elevated)
Urine Osmolality (normal 500 - 850)	Elevated - > 500	Elevated if oliguric; Lower if diuretic phase - < 350	< 350

Indications for Dialysis

» Easy acronym to remember reasons:

A: Acid/base imbalance

E: Electrolyte imbalance (hyperkalemia, hypermagnesemia, hyperphosphatemia)

I: Intoxications (ODs/toxins)

O: Overload (fluid)

U: Uremic symptoms

Laboratory findings in ATN in need of RRT:

» BUN > 35

» Creatinine > 4 or, creatinine
climbing ≥ 1 point/day

» Uncompensated
metabolic acidosis

» Anemia

» Electrolyte imbalances

* Increased potassium (> 6.5),
magnesium, phosphate

* Decreased calcium, bicarb

* Abnormal urine electrolytes

» Uremic Syndrome symptoms
(when the BUN is elevated)

» Neurologic: Lethargy,
fatigue, seizures, coma

» Cardiovascular: ECG changes
(d/t hyperkalemia), signs of fluid
overload; tachycardia, S3 heart
sound, hypo/hypertension

» Hematologic: Anemia

» Pulmonary: Crackles,
pulmonary edema, SOB,
effusions, pleuritis from uremia

» Gastrointestinal: Decreased
appetite, nausea & vomiting,
ascites & fluid overload

General Treatment Goals for AKI

» Hemodynamic stability

» Improve renal perfusion

» Correct chemistry abnormalities
(electrolytes, BUN, creatinine)

» Monitor electrolyte imbalances

* During therapy

* After therapy

» Adequate hydration

* Careful use of diuretics

* Accurate, meticulous
daily weights

» Aggressive dialysis

» Monitor drug levels for toxicity

» Monitor coags

» Alter medication schedules
around dialysis if needed

» Modify medication
dosing—identify meds
cleared through kidneys

» Minimize exposure to
nephrotoxic medications

» Prevent infection

» Maintain nutritional state

Contrast induced nephropathy (CIN)

» Highest risk patients:

» Diabetics, HTN, heart failure

» Pre-existing renal insufficiency

» Dehydrated

» Concurrent use of nephrotoxic medications (i.e. NSAIDS, ACE Inhibitors)

» High volume of contrast

» 10% of all patients who receive contrast dye develop CIN—yikes!

» ***HYDRATION!!! is the key to prevention

* A little rhyme to remember: The **solution** to **pollution** (contrast dye) is **dilution**!!!!

* Hydrate to protect the kidneys!!!

» Sodium bicarbonate infusion—1 hour before & 6 hours after exposure to contrast dye

* Not much evidence to support this

» N-Acetylcysteine (Mucomyst) for prevention (stinky!)

* 600 mg PO day before & day of contrast exposure (total of 4 doses)

* Thought to prevent toxicity to renal tubules

* Not much evidence to support this

Chronic Kidney Disease (CKD)

» Slow, progressive deterioration of renal function

» Persistent & progressive reduction in GFR (< 60 ml/min/1.73 m^2) and/or albuminuria

» Diminished renal reserve puts patients at higher risk for development

Lab Findings:

» Anemia

» Increased BUN, creatinine, phosphate

» Decreased calcium, bicarb, protein

Risk Factors for the development of Chronic Kidney Disease (CKD)

- » Diabetes*
- » Hypertension*
- » Autoimmune diseases
- » Systemic infection
- » Urinary stones or strictures

- » Prolong exposure to nephrotoxic drugs
- » Elderly
- » Race or ethnic background
- » Exposure to chemicals or environmental toxins
- » Family history

*Together responsible for 70% of CRF cases

Stages of Chronic Kidney Disease—mostly FYI

- » **Stage 1:** Damage w/ increased GFR
  - (> 90 ml/min/1.73 m^2)
- » **Stage 2:** Mild reduction GFR
  - (60 – 89 ml/min/1.73 m^2)
- » **Stage 3:** Moderate reduction in GFR

- (30 – 59 ml/min/1.73 m^2)
- » **Stage 4:** Severe reduction in GFR
  - (15 – 29 ml/min/1.73 m^2)
- » **Stage 5:** Kidney Failure
  - (< 15 ml/min/1.73 m^2)

Dialysis

Emergent dialysis options:

- » Hemodialysis
- » Continuous renal replacement therapy (CRRT)
- » Peritoneal

Principles of Dialysis

» Two compartments (blood & filtrate) separated by a semi-permeable membrane

» Pressure gradients are created

» Water, toxins, electrolytes & drugs can cross the membrane

» Goal is to reach equilibrium on each side of the membrane

Hemodialysis

» Intermittent

» Slow Low Efficiency Dialysis (SLED)

  • HD at lower flow rate; usually over 12 hours

» Artificial kidney (hemofilter) with a synthetic membrane

» Dialysate is bicarbonate & sodium based with electrolytes

» Short term access

  • Double lumen catheter

» Long term access

  • AV fistula

Hemodialysis Complications

» Hypotension

» Dysrhythmias (d/t electrolyte shifts)

» Angina

» Fever from pyrogenic reaction

» Coagulopathy, thrombocytopenia

» Disequilibrium syndrome (post-treatment cerebral edema)

» Air embolism

Air Embolism

Venous signs:

» Shortness of breath

» Chest pain

» Acute right heart failure (if obstructs blood flow from right heart to the lungs)

» Looks like a pulmonary embolism!

Treatment:

» Lay on left side, trendelenburg position

» Hyperoxygenate with 100% FiO_2; accelerates the removal of nitrogen in the air embolism

» Hyperbaric chamber

Arterial signs:

» Change in LOC (looks like a stroke!)

» Decreased arterial flow and perfusion (looks like an occluded artery)

* It only takes 2 ml of air to be fatal in an artery
* Only 0.5 ml air to be fatal in a coronary artery

Continuous Renal Replacement Therapy (CRRT)

» Slow continuous fluid removal

» Used in patients who are hemodynamically unstable

» Must have sufficient mean arterial pressure (MAP) or AV gradient to run CRRT

* AV Gradient is calculated by using the MAP – CVP
* > 60 mm Hg is desired

» If the AV gradient is too low, vasopressors may be needed to increase the blood pressure

» Indications: fluid removal refractory to diuretics

Complications:

» Hypotension

» Bleeding (anticoagulation)

» Hypothermia—can use a warmer

» Filter/circuit clotting

» Membrane rupture (blood in effluent bag)

* Immediately stop treatment & disconnect!

CRRT modes

» Slow Continuous Ultrafiltration (SCUF)— removing excess fluid only

» Continuous venovenous hemofiltration (CVVH)

* with hemodialysis (CVVHD)

* with hemodiafiltration (CVVHDF)

» Continuous arteriovenous (CAVH/CAVHD/F)

Peritoneal Dialysis (PD)

» Primarily used for long term kidney failure, but can be used in emergencies

» Soft catheter inserted percutaneously into abdominal cavity

» Abdominal mesenteric capillary bed is utilized as the semi-permeable membrane

» Glucose-based dialysate is used

* 1.5%, 2.5%, 4.25% glucose solutions are often used

* 4.25% solution is going to pull more fluid off than 1.5%

* Higher glucose concentration = ↑ fluid removal (via diffusion gradient)

» Usually 2 Liter exchanges done every 3 - 4 hours

» Advantages: patient can do at home, cost effective, no need for anticoagulation or vascular access

Complications of Peritoneal Dialysis (PD):

» Peritonitis (increased WBCs, temperature derangements)

» Hyperglycemia

» Diaphragmatic pressure which can cause respiratory compromise

» Pleural effusions

» Visceral herniation or perforation

» Recent abdominal surgery

» Abdominal adhesions

» Peritonitis

Electrolyte Imbalances

Sodium

Functions:

» Regulates total body water

» Transmission of nerve impulses

» Regulation of acid-base balance

» Muscle contraction

Hypernatremia Na$^+$ > 145 mEq/L

Causes:

» Dehydration

» Excess administration
of NaCl or NaHCO$_3$

» Hypertonic enteral feedings

» Burn injury

Symptoms:

» Thirst, tachycardia, hypotension,
restless, irritable, lethargy,
muscle weakness, flushed skin,
oliguria (with dehydration)

» May also see increased
hematocrit (hemo-concentrated)

» Increased chloride

* Often > 106 mEq/L

» Increased serum osmolality

» Increased urine specific
gravity due to concentrated
urine in dehydration

* Often > 1.025

» Decreased urine Na$^+$

Treatment:

- » Fluid hydration

- » Free H_2O

- » Diuretics (to remove sodium)—of appropriate for cause

Hyponatremia—$Na^+ < 130$ mEq/L

Causes:

- » Excess H_2O or Na^+ depletion

- » Water retention

- » Dehydration

- » NG tube suction

- » SIADH—dilutional hyponatremia

- » Diarrhea

- » Intestinal surgery

- » DKA

Symptoms:

- » Neuro changes, headache, confusion, coma, death

- » Anxiety, weakness, abdominal cramping, seizures, hypotension, tachycardia, shock

Treatment:

- » Slow Na^+ correction!!!!
  - • No more than 12 mEq/day

- » Na^+ Phosphate 1 – 2 mmol/hour over 3 – 4 hours

- » Hypertonic saline

- » Na^+ tabs

Potassium

» Normal K^+ levels: 3.5 – 5.0 mEq/L

» 90% intracellular, 10% in serum

» Na^+/K^+ pump—maintains normal cell volume and electro-neutrality of the cell membrane

Functions of K^+:

» Transmission of nerve impulses

» Intracellular osmolality

» Enzymatic reactions

» Acid-base balance

» Myocardial, skeletal & smooth muscle contractility

Potassium Regulation

» Kidneys—Primary excretory source

  • So efficient rarely have hyper states in normal renal function

• In the presence of aldosterone, K^+ is excreted by the renal tubules

» Intestines—excrete K^+

Hypokalemia: K^+ < 3.5 mEq/L

Causes:

» Increased loss

» GI: Vomiting, NGT suctioning (aggravated by metabolic alkalosis)

» Diarrhea, fistula, ileostomy

» Excessive urinary loss

» Hyperaldosterone states, thiazide diuretics, amphotericin, gentamycin, cisplatin

» Inadequate intake

» Anorexia, ETOH

» Magnesium depletion

» Insulin

Symptoms:

» Clinical presentation—develop symptoms when $K^+ < 3.0$ mEq/L

» Cardiovascular irritability

   • Ventricular irritability (PVCs) $K^+ < 3.2$

» Ventricular fibrillation

» Depressed ST segment

» Development of a u-wave

» Prolonged QT interval

» Potentates digoxin activity

» Muscle cramping

» Intracellular shift causing Alka-*LO*-sis

   • 0.1 unit ↑ in pH, causes ↓ K^+ by 0.4 mEq/L

Treatment:

» Replace K^+

» Oral supplements or increased dietary intake when possible

» IV - Standard dose 10 - 20 mEq over 1 - 2 hours

   • Central line administration preferred

» Eliminate or treat conditions that promote K^+ shifts (i.e. alkalosis)

» Ensure adequate renal function

Hyperkalemia - $K^+ > 5.5$ mEq

Causes:

» Renal failure (~75% of all cases)

   • Inability of renal tubules to excrete K^+

» Acidosis

» Decreased cardiac output

» Elderly taking K^+ sparing diuretics

» Severe trauma & burns

» Infection

» Addison's disease

» Increased consumption of table salt or antacids

Symptoms:

» Nausea & vomiting

» Diarrhea

» Tingling skin

» Numbness in hands & feet

» Flaccid paralysis

» Apathy, confusion

Cardiac symptoms:

» Tall tented symmetrical T waves ($K^+ > 6.5$)

» Widened QRS, prolonged PR, widened P wave ($K^+ > 8.0$)

» Decreased automaticity (K^+ 10 - 11.0)

» P waves disappear

» QRS merges with T to form sine wave

» Asystole or ventricular fibrillation

» Decreased strength of cardiac contraction

Treatment:

» Emergency (move potassium):

• Regular Insulin

▷ Dextrose if normal or low glucose to prevent hypoglycemia

• Calcium chloride (cardiac protectant; no effect on K^+ levels)

• $NaHCO_3$—not as efficient as insulin

• Nebulized albuterol

▷ Onset ~15 min., duration about 15 – 90 min.

» Remove potassium:

• Dialysis

• Loop diuretics

• Sodium polystyrene sulfonate (Kayexalate)

▷ Dose 15 grams 1 - 4 doses/ day

▷ 24 hours to correct

▷ Shouldn't be used for emergent treatment

Magnesium

» Normal level 1.5 – 2.5 mEq/L

Functions:

» Neuromuscular transmission

» Cardiac contraction

» Activation of enzymes for cellular metabolism

» Active transport at the cellular level

» Transmission of hereditary info.

Hypomagnesemia - Mg^{++} < 1.4 mEq/L

Causes:

» Increased excretion

» NG suctioning, diarrhea, fistulas

» Diuretics: blocks Na^+ reabsorption

» Osmotic diuresis

» Antibiotics & anti-neoplastics

» Hypercalcemia, hypokalemia

» Decreased intake

» Chronic alcoholism

» Malabsorption

» Acute pancreatitis

Symptoms:

» CV: Tachycardia, depressed ST segment,

» Torsades de Pointes! Caused by prolonged QT!

  • Polymorphic ventricular tachycardia

» PACs & PVCs

» Hypotension

» Coronary artery spasm

» Neuromuscular

* Twitching, paresthesia, cramps, muscle tremors
* +Chvostek & Trousseau's signs
  ▷ twitching of face or hand

» CNS: mentation changes, seizures

» Hypokalemia

Treatment:

» Assess renal function

» Increase Mg^{++} intake

» Increased risk for digoxin toxicity

» Dietary: diet or PO supplementation
  * Add to IV or TPN

» $MgSO_4$ 1 - 2 grams IV over 60 minutes, emergency give over 1 - 2 minutes

* Monitor BP & airway when administering magnesium!
* Can get hypotensive & flushed with Mg^{++}

» Monitor neurological status

» Monitor K^+ and Ca^{++}

» Follow serial magnesium levels

Hypermagnesemia - Mg^{++} > 2.5 mEq/L

Causes:

» Decreased excretion from renal failure is the most common

» Can also see in acidosis, DKA

Symptoms:

» 3 - 5 mEq/L Peripheral dilation, facial flushing, hypotension

» 4 - 7 mEq/L Drowsiness, lethargy

» When Mg^{++} is elevated, patients get the "Mag Drag"! (Lethargy, drowsy)

Treatment:

» Increase excretion of Mg^{++}
by using fluids & diuretics

Hypocalcemia—Ca^{++} < 8.5

» Follow ionized (active) Ca^{++}

• Normal: 1.1 – 1.35 mmol/L

Causes:

» Diarrhea

» Diuretics

» Malabsorption

» Chronic renal failure

» Alkalosis; Ca^{++} bound to
albumin & is inactive

» Phosphate & calcium have
an inverse relationship
to each other!

Symptoms:

» CV: Prolonged QTc, ↓BP,
↓CO, ventricular ectopy,
ventricular fibrillation

» Neuromuscular: Tingling,
spasms, tetany, seizures

  • Twitching, paresthesia,
cramps, muscle tremors

  • +Chvostek & Trousseau's signs

» Respiratory: Bronchospasm;
labored shallow breathing

» Gastrointestinal: smooth
muscle hyperactivity

» Bleeding; Ca^{++} needed to clot

» Safety: confusion & seizures

» Muscle cramps can
precede tetany

Treatment:

» Administer calcium

Hypophosphatemia—PO$_4$ < 2.5 mg/dL

» Necessary for cellular energy

» Tissue catabolism: increase use in tissue repair

Causes:

» Decreased intake

» ETOH

» Small bowel disease

» Increased elimination

» Vomiting and diarrhea

» Use of phosphate binding antacids

» Increased urinary losses: osmotic diuresis, thiazide diuretics

» Increased utilization

» Intracellular shifts

» Alkalosis (respiratory)

» Refeeding syndrome
  * See when patient has been NPO & nutrition is restarted

Symptoms: (secondary to decreases in ATP & 2,3 DPG)

» Acute:
  * Confusion, seizures, coma
  * Chest pain due to poor oxygenation of the myocardium
  * Numbness and tingling of the fingers, circumoral region
  * Incoordination
  * Speech difficulty
  * Weakness of respiratory muscles

» Chronic:
  * Memory loss, lethargy
  * Bone pain
  * Hypomagnesemia

Treatment:

» Identification and elimination of the cause

» Increase dietary intake of phosphate

» Oral or IV phosphate supplements

- K^+ phosphate
- Na^+ phosphate

Hyperphosphatemia—PO$_4$ > 4.5 mg/dL

Causes:

» Increased intake from phosphate containing antacids

» Decreased excretion - renal failure

» Transcellular shifts

» Respiratory acidosis, intracellular release

» Cell lysis of RBC, skeletal muscle or tumor cells

Symptoms:

» Rebound hypocalcemia

» Phosphate binds with free calcium and ionized serum calcium falls

» Ectopic disposition of Ca-PO$_4$

» Anorexia, nausea, vomiting

» Muscle weakness, hyperreflexia, tetany

» Tachycardia

» ↑PO$_4$ =↓Ca^{++}

Treatment:

» Identification and elimination of cause

» Use of aluminum, magnesium or calcium gels or antacids: binds phosphorus in the gut

» Diet low in phosphorus

» Avoid meats, fish, poultry, milk, whole grains, seeds, nuts, eggs, dried beans

» Dialysis therapy

» Acetazolamide stimulated urinary PO_4 excretion

You can do it!

Synergy Review

AACN Blueprint for the Professional Caring & Ethical Practice portion of the CCRN® Exam

- Advocacy/Moral Agency
- Caring Practices
- Response to Diversity
- Facilitation of Learning
- Collaboration
- Systems Thinking
- Clinical Inquiry

Note: For this section I listed "big picture" ideas to keep in mind. I recommend doing practice questions to apply many of these concepts.

Advocacy & Moral Agency

» Working on another's behalf and representing concerns of patients, families and nursing staff (reference: AACN Synergy Model definition)

» Respecting patient's rights, beliefs and values

Basic rights:

» Informed decision making

» Education on disease process, treatments, plan of care

» Respect & honor patient's wishes & choices

» For healthcare providers to advocate and speak up on behalf of our patients

» Privacy of information

Multidisciplinary plan of care

» Involves the care team (physicians, nursing, respiratory, PT, OT, nutrition, social work) to set comprehensive expectations of the trajectory of care for the patient

Includes:

» Medications

» Tests

» Treatments

» Discharge needs

Benefits of a multidisciplinary approach:

» Reduced length of stay

» Better outcomes

» Better continuity of care

» Reduced costs

» Improved communication with the patient, family & teams

Advance Directives

» Used as a way for patients
to identify their wishes
at the end of life

  * They should be honored
    regardless of opposing
    family opinions

» Should identify a decision-maker
if patient is incapacitated and
unable to make decisions

» Consider Palliative Care
consult if appropriate

» Spiritual care to meet religious
needs of patient and family

» Facilitate any rituals
the patient/family are
requesting at end of life

» Ensure comfort

  * Outline plan with
    family/loved ones

Other thoughts:

» When communicating,
always be honest

» Do not contract with family
to be secretive about the
patient's diagnosis

» Do not withhold information
from the patient

» Always maintain confidentiality

» Use open communication

  * Ask "What is your understanding
    of the situation, disease
    state or treatment plan"?

» Keep the patient safe

» Resolve ethical & clinical
concerns in a non-
confrontational manner

» Consult the Ethics Committee
if unable to come to resolution

Core Patient Characteristics and Nurse Competencies as Defined in the Synergy Model

Advocacy and Moral Agency	Working on another's behalf and representing the concerns of the patient/family and nursing staff; serving as a moral agent in identifying and helping to resolve ethical and clinical concerns within and outside the clinical setting
Level 1	Works on behalf of patient; self-assesses personal values; aware of ethical conflicts/issues that may surface in clinical setting; makes ethical/moral decisions based on rules; represents patient when patient cannot represent self; aware of patients' rights
Level 3	Works on behalf of patient and family; considers patient values and incorporates in care, even when differing from personal values; supports colleagues in ethical and clinical issues; moral decision-making can deviate from rules; demonstrates give and take with patient's family, allowing them to speak/represent themselves when possible; aware of patient and family rights
Level 5	Works on behalf of patient, family and community; advocates from patient/family perspective, whether similar to or different from personal values; advocates ethical conflict and issues from patient/family perspective; suspends rules—patient and family drive moral decision-making; empowers the patient and family to speak for/represent themselves; achieves mutuality within patient/professional relationships

Caring Practices

» Minimize safety risks
to the patient

  * Communicate and speak
    up immediately if there is
    a risk or safety issue!

» Ensure the environment is safe
and comfortable for the patient

» Ensure patient understands
the plan of care

» Identify what the patient and/
or family sees as a priority
in their plan of care

» Identify a spokesperson
to contact with updates

» Ensure families are updated
on the patient's status

» Goal is always to develop
trust with family

» Assess the families coping
needs and support them

» Families are at risk for
PTSD as well as patients

» Make sure the patient and
family understands expectations
around visiting policies

  * How many people can
    visit at one time?

  * Age restrictions?

  * Is there flexibility?

» The ideal situation/policy is
open visitation tailored to
the patient's wants & needs

» Consider providing written
information regarding
visiting policies

  * Include unit routines

  * Shift change expectations/rules

» Family presence during
resuscitation and high
risk procedures is widely
accepted across the country

» If family is present during
CPR, ensure someone can
stay with them for support
(i.e. spiritual care, a nurse)

» Keep the environment quiet

  * Control lights and noise
    as much as possible

  * Promote sleep

  * Provide eye masks and ear plugs

  * Adjust nuisance alarms
    from monitors

» Consider alternative
therapies as appropriate

  * Pet therapy, music therapy,
    aromatherapy, massage

Core Patient Characteristics and Nurse Competencies as Defined in the Synergy Model

Caring Practices	Nursing activities that create a compassionate, supportive and therapeutic environment for patients and staff, with the aim of promoting comfort and healing and preventing unnecessary suffering. Includes, but is not limited to, vigilance, engagement and responsiveness of caregivers, including family and healthcare personnel
Level 1	Focuses on the usual and customary needs of the patient; no anticipation of future needs; bases care on standards and protocols; maintains a safe physical environment; acknowledges death as a potential outcome
Level 3	Responds to subtle patient and family changes; engages with the patient as a unique patient in a compassionate manner; recognizes and tailors caring practices to the individuality of patient and family; domesticates the patient's and family's environment; recognizes that death may be an acceptable outcome
Level 5	Has astute awareness and anticipates patient and family changes and needs; fully engaged with and sensing how to stand alongside the patient, family and community; caring practices follow the patient and family lead; anticipates hazards and avoids them, and promotes safety throughout patient's and family's transitions along the healthcare continuum; orchestrates the process that ensures patient's/family's comfort and concerns surrounding issues of death and dying are met

Data from: American Association of Critical-Care Nurses. The AACN Synergy Model for Patient Care. Aliso Viejo, CA: AACN. http://www.aacn.org/WD/Certifications/Content/synmodel.content?menu=Certification. Accessed August 25, 2016

Response to Diversity

» Make every effort to meet the ethical, religious and cultural needs of your patient

» Cultural sensitivity—be aware of differences that may impact clinical care

» Incorporate the patient's values into care as much as possible

» Avoid stereotypes of cultures and race

» Modify care to meet the patient's needs

» Pain may be expressed differently based on culture

» Maintain patient privacy

» Consider dietary needs based on cultural differences (i.e. vegetarian, no beef or pork)

Core Patient Characteristics and Nurse Competencies as Defined in the Synergy Model

Response to Diversity	The sensitivity to recognize, appreciate and incorporate differences into the provision of care; differences may include, but are not limited to, cultural differences, spiritual beliefs, gender, race, ethnicity, lifestyle, socioeconomic status, age and values
Level 1	Assesses cultural diversity; provides care based on own belief system; learns the culture of the healthcare environment
Level 3	Inquires about cultural differences and considers their impact on care; accommodates personal and professional differences in the plan of care; helps patient/family understand the culture of the healthcare system
Level 5	Responds to, anticipates and integrates cultural differences into patient/family care; appreciates and incorporates differences, including alternative therapies, into care; tailors healthcare culture, to the extent possible, to meet the diverse needs and strengths of the patient/family

Data from: American Association of Critical-Care Nurses. The AACN Synergy Model for Patient Care. Aliso Viejo, CA: AACN. http://www.aacn.org/WD/Certifications/Content/synmodel.content?menu=Certification. Accessed August 25, 2016

Facilitation of Learning

Staff Educational Needs

» If you have not been trained to care for certain patients or devices/treatments they are receiving, you should not accept that assignment or agree to cover for breaks

» Notify the charge nurse immediately to be assigned to a different patient

» You must meet the competencies to care for patients with specialized needs (i.e. ECMO, IABP, PA catheter)

Patient & Family Educational Needs

» Teach back method—have them show you how to do a skill vs. telling them how to do it

» Provide ongoing education if needed

» Provide episodic education based on learning needs

» Do not wait until discharge to provide all teaching at once

» Repeat and reinforce the information and assesses for knowledge deficits

» Specialty consults for specific educational needs (i.e. heart failure, diabetic education)

» Identify barriers to learning (i.e. cognitive, language) and re-strategize educational plans

» If there is a language barrier, consult a medical interpreter

  • Families or friends should not be used to interpret medical information

» Avoid medical jargon and terminology as much as possible

Core Patient Characteristics and Nurse Competencies as Defined in the Synergy Model

Facilitation of Learning	The ability to facilitate learning for patients/families, nursing staff, other members of the healthcare team and community; includes both formal and informal facilitation of learning
Level 1	Follows planned educational programs; sees patient/family education as a separate task from delivery of care; provides data without seeking to assess patient's readiness or understanding; has limited knowledge of the totality of the educational needs; focuses on a nurse's perspective; sees the patient as a passive recipient
Level 3	Adapts planned educational programs; begins to recognize and integrate different ways of teaching into delivery of care; incorporates patient's understanding into practice; sees the overlapping of educational plans from different healthcare providers' perspectives; begins to see the patient as having input into goals; begins to see individualism
Level 5	Creatively modifies or develops patient/family education programs; integrates patient/family education throughout delivery of care; evaluates patient's understanding by observing behavior changes related to learning; is able to collaborate and incorporate all healthcare providers' and educational plans into the patient/family educational program; sets patient-driven goals for education; sees patient/family as having choices and consequences that are negotiated in relation to education

Data from: American Association of Critical-Care Nurses. The AACN Synergy Model for Patient Care. Aliso Viejo, CA: AACN. http://www.aacn.org/WD/Certifications/Content/synmodel.content?menu=Certification. Accessed August 25, 2016

Collaboration

» Make referrals as needed for other multidisciplinary services

  * Example: If you patient is high risk for skin breakdown, consult with Physical Therapy & Nutrition

» Include family as much as appropriate in planning and patient care

» Include patients and families in multidisciplinary rounds as much as possible

» Prepare patients and families for transitions in care as early as possible

  * Transfer to another unit or facility

» If the patient is transferring to another unit or facility, encourage the family to tour the new location prior to transfer

  * This may reduce fear and anxiety

  * Consider having the unit charge nurse or manager meet the patient and family prior to discharge

» If discharging, assess resources available for patient

  * Consult social work or appropriate groups for gaps in resources

Core Patient Characteristics and Nurse Competencies as Defined in the Synergy Model

Collaboration	Working with others (e.g., patients, families, healthcare providers) in a way that promotes/encourages each person's contributions toward achieving optimal/realistic patient/family goals; involves intra- and inter-disciplinary work with colleagues and community
Level 1	Willing to be taught, coached and/or mentored; participates in team meetings and discussions regarding patient care and/or practice issues; open to various team members' contributions
Level 3	Seeks opportunities to be taught, coached and/or mentored; elicits others' advice and perspectives; initiates and participates in team meetings and discussions regarding patient care and/or practice issues; recognizes and suggests various team members' participation
Level 5	Seeks opportunities to teach, coach and mentor and to be taught, coached and mentored; facilitates active involvement and complementary contributions of others in team meetings and discussions regarding patient care and/or practice issues; involves/recruits diverse resources when appropriate to optimize patient outcomes

Data from: American Association of Critical-Care Nurses. The AACN Synergy Model for Patient Care. Aliso Viejo, CA: AACN. http://www.aacn.org/WD/Certifications/Content/synmodel.content?menu=Certification. Accessed August 25, 2016

Systems Thinking

Patient Safety

» If a mistake is made, do not try to cover it up

» Talk to the patient and family about what happened

» Apologize for the mistake

» Explain the plan for follow up

» If a mistake is made, always assess for system issues

» Consider participating in a hospital committee to better understand system issues

» Maintain a non-punitive environment to support healthcare providers

General rules:

» Avoid unapproved abbreviations

» Always use 2 person identifiers

* Name, Medical Record Number, DOB

Core Patient Characteristics and Nurse Competencies as Defined in the Synergy Model

Systems Thinking	Body of knowledge and tools that allow the nurse to manage whatever environmental and system resources exist for the patient/family and staff, within or across healthcare and non-healthcare systems
Level 1	Uses a limited array of strategies; limited outlook—sees the pieces or components; does not recognize negotiation as an alternative; sees patient and family within the isolated environment of the unit; sees self as key resource
Level 3	Develops strategies based on needs and strengths of patient/family; able to make connections within components; sees opportunity to negotiate, but may not have strategies; developing a view of the patient/family transition process; recognizes how to obtain resources beyond self
Level 5	Develops, integrates and applies a variety of strategies that are driven by the needs and strengths of the patient/family; global or holistic outlook—sees the whole rather than the pieces; knows when and how to negotiate and navigate through the system on behalf of patients and families; anticipates needs of patients and families as they move through the healthcare system; utilizes untapped and alternative resources as necessary

Data from: American Association of Critical-Care Nurses. The AACN Synergy Model for Patient Care. Aliso Viejo, CA: AACN. http://www.aacn.org/WD/Certifications/Content/synmodel.content?menu=Certification. Accessed August 25, 2016

Clinical Inquiry

Evidence-Based Practice (EBP)

» Understanding of what the best, most reliable evidence is to provide a standard of care for patients

» Don't practice on the idea of "That's the way we've always done it"

» If there is a need for a change in practice:

  • Collaborate with multidisciplinary team

  • Conduct a literature review

• Randomized-controlled trials would be highest level of evidence

• Systematic reviews and meta-analysis are very helpful

• Consider national practice guidelines from professional organizations (i.e. American Heart Association, Surviving Sepsis Campaign)

» Establish a unit-based council

» Create an environment of inquiry

Core Patient Characteristics and Nurse Competencies as Defined in the Synergy Model

Clinical Judgment	Clinical reasoning, which includes clinical decision-making, critical thinking and a global grasp of the situation, coupled with nursing skills acquired through a process of integrating formal and informal experiential knowledge and evidence-based guidelines
Level 1	Collects basic-level data; follows algorithms, decision trees and protocols with all populations and is uncomfortable deviating from them; matches formal knowledge with clinical events to make decisions; questions the limits of one's ability to make clinical decisions and delegates the decision-making to other clinicians; includes extraneous detail
Level 3	Collects and interprets complex patient data; makes clinical judgments based on an immediate grasp of the whole picture for common or routine patient populations; recognizes patterns and trends that may predict the direction of illness; recognizes limits and seeks appropriate help; focuses on key elements of case, while sorting out extraneous details

Level 5	Synthesizes and interprets multiple, sometimes conflicting, sources of data; makes judgment based on an immediate grasp of the whole picture, unless working with new patient populations; uses past experiences to anticipate problems; helps patient and family see the "big picture"; recognizes the limits of clinical judgment and seeks multidisciplinary collaboration and consultation with comfort; recognizes and responds to the dynamic situation

Data from: American Association of Critical-Care Nurses. The AACN Synergy Model for Patient Care. Aliso Viejo, CA: AACN. http://www.aacn.org/WD/Certifications/Content/synmodel.content?menu=Certification. Accessed August 25, 2016

Core Patient Characteristics and Nurse Competencies as Defined in the Synergy Model

Clinical Inquiry	The ongoing process of questioning and evaluating practice and providing informed practice; creating practice changes through research utilization and experiential learning
Level 1	Follows standards and guidelines; implements clinical changes and research-based practices developed by others; recognizes the need for further learning to improve patient care; recognizes obvious changing patient situation (e.g., deterioration, crisis); needs and seeks help to identify patient problem
Level 3	Questions appropriateness of policies and guidelines; questions current practice; seeks advice, resources or information to improve patient care; begins to compare and contrast possible alternatives
Level 5	Improves, deviates from or individualizes standards and guidelines for particular patient situations or populations; questions and/or evaluates current practice based on patients' responses, review of the literature, research and education/learning; acquires knowledge and skills needed to address questions arising in practice and improve patient care; (The domains of clinical judgment and clinical inquiry converge at the expert level; they cannot be separated)

Data from: American Association of Critical-Care Nurses. The AACN Synergy Model for Patient Care. Aliso Viejo, CA: AACN. http://www.aacn.org/WD/Certifications/Content/synmodel.content?menu=Certification. Accessed August 25, 2016

Legal/Ethical Principles

Beneficence:

» The action that is done for the benefit of others

» Beneficent actions can be taken to help prevent or remove harms or to simply improve the situation of others

Nonmaleficence:

» "Do no harm"

» Refrain from providing ineffective treatments or acting with malice toward patients

• Offers little useful guidance to physicians since many beneficial therapies also have serious risks

» Pertinent ethical issue is whether the benefits outweigh the burdens

Veracity:

» Principle of truth telling, and it is grounded in respect for persons and the concept of autonomy

Justice:

» The fair distribution of benefits and burdens

Paternalism:

» What is best for patients may affect the decisions they make about their patient's diagnosis, prognosis or therapy

» The nurse may choose to withhold information from the patient and family members

» The interference with a person's liberty of action justified by reason referring exclusively to the welfare of the person being coerced

Fidelity:

» Dedication, loyalty, truthfulness, advocacy and fairness to patients

Confidentiality:

» The obligation of professionals **who have access to patient records or communication to hold that information in confidence**

Utilitarianism:

» To promote the greatest good that is possible in situations

You can do it!

Core Patient Characteristics and Nurse Competencies as Defined in the Synergy Model

Patient Characteristics	Description
Resiliency	**The capacity to return to a restorative level of functioning using compensatory/coping mechanisms; the ability to bounce back quickly after an insult**
Level 1—Minimally resilient	Unable to mount a response; failure of compensatory/ coping mechanisms; minimal reserves; brittle
Level 3—Moderately resilient	Able to mount a moderate response; able to initiate some degree of compensation; moderate reserves
Level 5—Highly resilient	Able to mount and maintain a response; intact compensatory/coping mechanisms; strong reserves; endurance
Vulnerability	**Susceptibility to actual or potential stressors that may adversely affect patient outcomes**
Level 1—Highly vulnerable	Susceptible; unprotected, fragile
Level 3—Moderately vulnerable	Somewhat susceptible; somewhat protected
Level 5—Minimally vulnerable	Safe; out of the woods; protected, not fragile
Stability	**The ability to maintain a steady-state equilibrium**
Level 1—Minimally stable	Labile; unstable; unresponsive to therapies; high risk of death
Level 3—Moderately stable	Able to maintain steady state for limited period of time; some responsiveness to therapies
Level 5—Highly stable	Constant; responsive to therapies; low risk of death
Complexity	**The intricate entanglement of two or more systems (e.g., body, family, therapies)**
Level 1—Highly complex	Intricate; complex patient/family dynamics; ambiguous/ vague; atypical presentation
Level 3—Moderately complex	Moderately involved patient/family dynamics
Level 5—Minimally complex	Straightforward; routine patient/family dynamics; simple/ clear cut; typical presentation

Resource availability	Extent of resources (e.g., technical, fiscal, personal, psychological and social) the patient/family/community bring to the situation
Level 1—Few resources	Necessary knowledge and skills not available; necessary financial support not available; minimal personal/psychological supportive resources; few social systems resources
Level 3—Moderate resources	Limited knowledge and skills available; limited financial support available; limited personal/psychological supportive resources; limited social systems resources
Level 5—Many resources	Extensive knowledge and skills available and accessible; financial resources readily available; strong personal/psychological supportive resources; strong social systems resources
Participation in care	**Extent to which patient/family engages in aspects of care**
Level 1—No participation	Patient and family unable or unwilling to participate in care
Level 3—Moderate level of participation	Patient and family need assistance in care
Level 5—Full participation	Patient and family fully able to participate in care
Participation in decision-making	**Extent to which patient/family engages in decision-making**
Level 1—No participation	Patient and family have no capacity for decision-making; requires surrogacy
Level 3—Moderate level of participation	Patient and family have limited capacity; seeks input/advice from others in decision-making
Level 5—Full participation	Patient and family have capacity, and makes decision for self
Predictability	**A characteristic that allows one to expect a certain course of events or course of illness**
Level 1—Not predictable	Uncertain; uncommon patient population/illness; unusual or unexpected course; does not follow critical pathway, or no critical pathway developed
Level 3—Moderately predictable	Wavering; occasionally noted patient population/illness
Level 5—Highly predictable	Certain; common patient population/illness; usual and expected course; follows critical pathway

About the author...

Nicole Kupchik has practiced as a Critical Care nurse for over twenty years. She obtained a Nursing Degree from Purdue University in 1993 and a Master of Nursing from the University of Washington in 2008.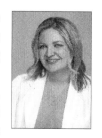

Nicole's nursing career began in the Chicago area. From 1995 to 1998, she journeyed across the United States as a traveling nurse, after which she landed in Seattle. Her first job in Seattle was in the Cardiothoracic Intensive Care Unit (5 SE) at the University of Washington. In 2001, she began working at Harborview Medical Center—a change that spurred an interest in resuscitation.

Shortly thereafter, Nicole was part of a multidisciplinary team that was one of the first in the United States to implement therapeutic hypothermia after cardiac arrest. As part of this effort, Nicole was responsible for protocol development and has published numerous papers on this topic.

In 2008, Nicole was part of a team that implemented a formalized Sepsis program at Harborview Medical Center. The program resulted in a reduction in mortality, hospital length of stay and a significant cost avoidance. She collaborated with IT specialists to develop innovative methods to electronically screen hospitalized patients in acute care units for sepsis. For this work, the program was awarded two Patient Safety & Clinical Leadership awards.

In 2002, Nicole obtained certification as a CCRN®. She admittedly attended three certification review courses before finally taking the exam! Once she passed the exam she questioned why she hesitated and lacked confidence to sit the exam. Shortly thereafter, Nicole began teaching segments of CCRN® certification review courses at her hospital. In 2006, she started co-teaching courses nationally.

Currently, she works as a staff nurse at Harborview Medical Center in Seattle, WA. She holds certification as a CCNS®, CCRN®, PCCN® & CMC®. In 2013, Nicole founded Nicole Kupchik Consulting & Education. She frequently teaches review courses nationally.

Today her courses are well attended and often sell out! Her wit and sense of humor make the course interesting & entertaining. Nicole has a gift of being able to break information down in a way that is really easy to understand. She hopes to instill confidence in attendees that they can do it!

OTHER BOOKS BY NICOLE KUPCHIK

Ace the CCRN®: You can do it! Practice Review Questions
Ace the PCCN®: You can do it! Study Guide
Ace the PCCN®: You can do it! Practice Review Questions

TO CONTACT NICOLE:

nicole@nicolekupchikconsulting.com

www.nicolekupchikconsulting.com

Nicole Kupchik Consulting and Education

You can do it!

Made in the USA
San Bernardino, CA
05 October 2018